LIFE *with* ME

LIFE *with* ME

WORDS OF WARRIORS

HAYLEY GREEN

This book is dedicated to every single ME sufferer out there.

For the daily battle you face fighting this illness, and the admirable strength you no doubt have.

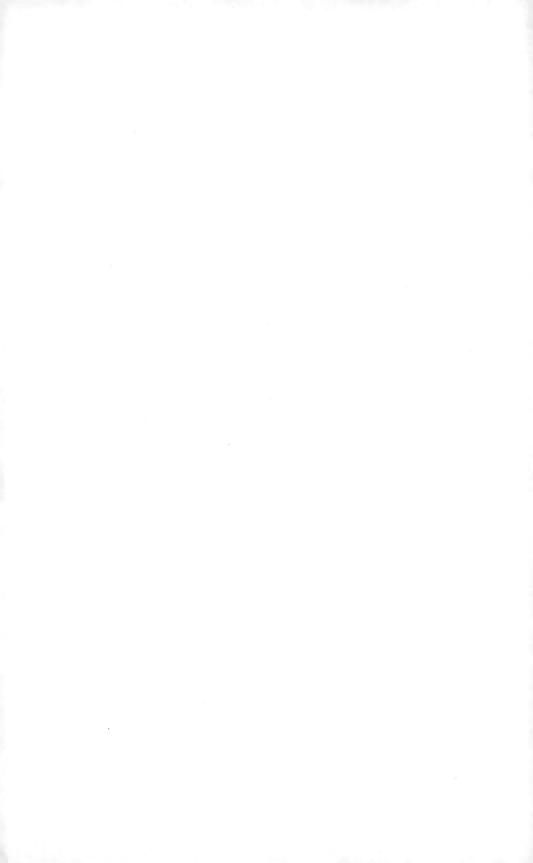

CONTENTS

ACKNOWLEDGMENTS

Thank you to everyone who was able to take the time and energy to contribute to this book.

The book aims to raise awareness, and 100% royalties are to be donated to Invest In ME, an independent charity campaigning for bio-medical research into the illness.

Thank you for making this happen.

INTRODUCTION

Here in the United Kingdom, there are around 250,000 ME (Myalgic Encephalomyelitis) sufferers.

The illness is severely debilitating and every person with the condition is fighting a daily battle. A battle to survive. A battle to be acknowledged. A battle for proper medical treatment.

The worst affected are bedbound, on oxygen, and tube fed. The disease has stolen years from people of all ages, even children, with no end in sight.

It can also be fatal, yet the illness receives very little government funding. This book aims to raise awareness into a very serious, neurological disease.

LIFE WITH *Hayley*

It crept on rather insidiously. I was in my early twenties when I began to feel extremely run down. I was catching every virus going, including Swine flu, which made me very ill.

I was working full time and going straight home to bed after an eight hour day. I didn't think too much of it, I had a busy social life and assumed that I was burning the candle at both ends. This is how it carried on for some time. I started making mistakes at work, and couldn't understand why I was feeling so 'out of it'. In 2011 I had started a new job as a sales representative. Although rewarding, it was a stressful role, and it wore me down. I then caught tonsillitis and was signed off work for two weeks. Soon the virus went, but weeks on I was still extremely wiped out. I knew something was wrong.

After several trips to the doctors I was diagnosed with ME. I was told there was 'no cure' and sent on my way. I was signed off again and eventually my employer was getting restless. I went back to work for a few days, but couldn't function. My head hurt, I was exhausted and my body ached. I was sent home. I then made the hard decision to hand in my notice due to poor health. I simply couldn't handle the pressure, and I wasn't getting any better.

A few months later I was referred to a specialist ME Clinic, where I was diagnosed with moderate ME by a specialist. I then attended a 6 week management course at the clinic. Whilst there we learnt about how ME developed, along with strategies for managing it such as rest and pacing.

Pacing, I soon learnt, helped. I also learnt that stress was a huge trigger for relapses. I had a long journey of 'boom and bust', and paying for over-exertion before I really learnt to pace myself. Although I had learnt how to manage the illness, I was still badly affected and by this stage mainly housebound. Since then, I have made some progress with the fatigue – I know my limits and although I still push past them at times, I am aware of what will make me worse, and do my best to avoid it.

I am now around 80-90% housebound, I rarely feel well enough to go out – and when I do, my symptoms are worse when I get home. Brightly lit and noisy environments such as supermarkets sap my energy and make me feel terribly unwell, so I have to avoid them.

I can't walk far without an increase in symptoms and when I over-do it I have to rest in bed to recover. This can take days or even weeks depending on how much I have done. I never wake up feeling refreshed; I am just as fatigued as when I get to bed. Most days I get intense pain in my muscles and joints, and sometimes this pain wakes me up during the night. I struggle with cognitive functions – word finding, remembering things and keeping up with a conversation.

When I am crashing, I go a deathly pale. I start slurring my words and feel intense vertigo and nausea. This is when I have to go to bed because if I continue what I am doing, it's a very fast, slippery slope.

I go out at every opportunity, which isn't often. When I do go out I have to rest in the days beforehand, and the days afterwards. I do have 'better' patches, where I think I am starting to recover, and then it hits me like a brick wall. Symptoms return as intense as ever. I wish I could do little things that many people (and I used to) take for granted. Popping to the shop for a pint of milk, long days out, food shopping (yes I actually miss this!), going out at the drop of a hat for a meal or quick drink – all of these things I can no longer do without planning and pacing, if I can do them at all.

I manage my illness well, making an effort to stay positive. I have every faith that one day I will recover from this dreadful disease. But for now, this is my reality.

LIFE WITH *Joanne*

Exuberant. A girl who was full of life, full of strength and vitality. A girl whose nickname was Duracell because of the amount of energy she once had. A girl who loved swimming and was called 'a mermaid in the water'. A girl who loved to walk miles through the fields with her dog. A girl who was a go getter, extremely active, a people person involved in everything going.

From achieving a degree in theology, to being in full swing with everything going on at my local church. A youth leader, GB officer, a soloist, involved in every outreach programme there was. A girl who gave up any holidays she had to do children's camps in the summer. A girl who worked full time every day and was out most nights at church. Once upon a time that girl was me.

Now I can no longer participate in any of the activities that I named. Why? What would cause an active person to just stop? To waste away? Depression? No!!! A very real physical illness called ME.

My once unstoppable body started to get ill the year after my degree. I was constantly weak and tired. I was fainting so often. I remember being rushed to hospital in an ambulance because once during a fainting episode they couldn't get me to come round. I was unconscious for what seemed like ages to observers. I started to get every infection under the sun. I was constantly on anti - biotics for chest, throat, kidney, ear infections. I constantly felt like I had the flu. Shivery, nauseous, achy. I saw doctors during this time but every blood test came back clear. So I battled on. I went to work every day and continued to live. But it was a massive struggle. I didn't know what was wrong with me. I just knew I felt like I was constantly fighting a body that didn't want to work. Work became a nightmare.

The fatigue and weakness grew worse, recurrent infections kept coming, my body felt so achy and sleep completely disappeared. I felt like I wasn't taken seriously by doctor. He had no answers but I knew I was getting sicker...

Then one day just after work I was at a friend's house eating Chinese food and I collapsed on her floor. Fainting was common for me but this time my body never recovered after that faint. I was left bedbound for four months.

It was during this time that a different doctor diagnosed ME. I finally had a label for the mystery illness but by this stage I was twenty-four years old and had been running to doctors with the nightmare symptoms for three years before I got an answer. I really believe that if my condition had been caught early and rest had been prescribed that I wouldn't still be ill today. That was eight years ago. I've lost all of my twenties to this illness and now I'm losing my thirties.

The eight years that have passed have been extremely difficult. I am mostly housebound. I go long periods of time unable to do anything for myself. I've had long periods of being carried to the bathroom, being bed bathed, and unable to lift a glass of water. My mother is my carer. I've had other spells where I can leave the house and go somewhere but after two hours out my body shrivels up with exhaustion and I suffer for any exertion.

What troubles me is that most health care professionals treat ME like they would depression: Anti-depressants, referrals for counselling, Cognitive Behaviour Therapy, and gentle exercise therapy. It's not just doctors. Most people seem to believe that ME is an 'All in the head' disease, with sufferers constantly being told 'You don't look sick' on our rare good days out. But why? Who in their right mind would want to go from being the active, exuberant person who walked and swam to this housebound, dependent woman in her early thirties? I have done everything in my power over the past 8 years to be an overcomer and not be overcome by this nightmare illness. I am a Christian and the Lord really helps me to get through every day and find purpose.

Encouragement is something I can do from a sickbed.

I wrote a book in 2010 and had it published - *A Myrtle Tree For Life's Briars*. It's about my journey with illness, written with the aim to bring comfort and hope to others. (Still available from me or amazon.) Through its sales I raised £3500 for an orphanage in Romania for abused, hurting and abandoned girls. In 2011 I sold jewellery to raise money for an organisation called 'Beauty for Ashes' which seeks to rescue young girls who have been sold into prostitution. I've found writing poetry for special events like births, weddings, anniversaries etc. to be something I can do. This year, 2014, I cut off my really long hair and donated it to the 'Little Princess Trust' to make wigs for sick children who've lost their hair to chemo and raised £1500 for the charity.

I am not my illness. I am still Joanne, though not the active Joanne I want to be and yearn with everything within me to be. I have tried with all that's within me to not let my limits limit me but to find ways to make my life count from bed. A quote by the poet Emily Dickinson keeps me going: 'If I can stop one heart from breaking I shall not live in vain.'

I'm determined to not become self-focused just because life hasn't gone my way. I do yearn for a cure. I yearn to be free. I yearn for doctors to stop treating a physical illness as a mental one. I yearn for answers and solutions not judgements and criticisms. I want to be the girl I was once upon a time. Until then, I will do my best to not let this illness kill my spirit and reach beyond my four walls to others who hurt.

LIFE WITH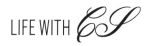

Before I developed ME, I was a wife and mother of three, a grandmother too. I ran my home which also had three dogs and two cats, did all my shopping, helped out at church where I was a regular attender and was extremely fit and active. One day in August 1985 I caught a virus that was going around the town, laying people very low. I went back to things too quickly and crashed again. This became a pattern, regularly being too exhausted to do the usual things. Within a year my failing marriage was over and I had to cope with working in this condition.

It wasn't good, in bed every weekend trying to recover from 21 hours a week of clerical work. Then I had a hysterectomy that went wrong and left me very ill and incapable of working. After some time I went back into education as I wasn't well enough to cope with physical work and had no qualifications. After some years I had an honours degree but then was too ill to continue with my PhD. Since then my health has deteriorated more and more and I am now housebound to a large degree, only going out for various appointments: doctors, hospital, etc.

I have never had an official diagnosis of ME as no doctor I have seen appears to know anything about it. In the early days a friend, a former nurse at the Royal Free Hospital, was sure it was Royal Free Disease, which I later learned to call ME. An assortment of blood tests, heart tests, and so forth have revealed nothing, of course. One specialist I saw just kept asking if I was depressed. Another refused to test for Lyme disease as he said, and I quote, 'The more you look for the more you tend to find.' Silly me, I thought that was the whole point!

I have most of the known symptoms of ME and have just become more and more unable to live any kind of normal life but I don't bother doctors about it. I am seventy years old now with osteoarthritis and high blood pressure, which isn't helping, and other complaints which I just put up with. I use mostly herbal supplements rather than drugs, which I tend to have bad reactions to. I have developed various other complaints over the years that don't make life any easier, including a rare tumour four years ago, successfully removed.

I now have eleven grandchildren and four great grandchildren, most of whom I never see. I can't cope with travel and they are scattered around the country, and very busy people. I see my daughter a couple of times a year and I have made friends online. The internet is now my lifeline to the outside world and I have self-published virtual books as a hobby which keeps me sane; as does my undimmed whacky sense of humour.

LIFE WITH *Charlotte Cann*

Before I was diagnosed I was at a point in my life where I felt like I was becoming independent. I was working full time in a job I enjoyed, I studied at college, I'd bought a car and was about to learn to drive, I was in a long term relationship and had wonderful family and friends. Life seemed to be going in the right direction and I was looking forward to the future. I'd got through a lot at a young age and I felt strong.

Then I began needing to sleep more and more; I'd crash on my bed as soon as I got back from work. One day I was working and suddenly I couldn't stay awake at my desk. My manager noticed and asked me to take a break, so I bought an energy drink thinking I was just tired, but knowing I'd been sleeping a lot. The drink didn't even touch it and she asked me to get checked out by a doctor. I had every blood test you can imagine, but no answers.

In the end I went private to see a consultant who told me straight away I had all of the symptoms of ME. and I had to quit my job right away, because otherwise I'd never improve and become permanently bed bound.

I was seventeen at that point, and what I'd just been told made me feel like my life was over.

Everything I had worked so hard for had gone up in smoke within a matter of minutes. The worst part for me is that not only is there no cure, but there is barely any help available. Most doctors don't seem to understand that ME is a serious neurological condition. I've had doctors tell me to smile, be positive and it will go away. Except this pain, this fatigue, everything that comes with ME isn't in my head, it's physical, and it's real. Doctors don't like patients with chronic health conditions because they can't fix it. There's no magic pill that will make you right as rain in a few weeks' time.

ME has cost me my job, my college course, my car, most of my friends, and a long term relationship. I'm lucky enough to be in another relationship now but it's not a standard young person's relationship. He is also my carer. I have to rely on him for most of my food and drink, sometimes even helping me to shower or go to the toilet. It's not glamorous; in fact it's very far from it. I'm eighteen years old now and the fact that I'm unable to look after myself eats away at me. I cry because of the pain and my boyfriend cries because he can't help me. This illness has taken so much from me but I try my best to remain positive. I take it one day at a time and try to live my life whenever I can. If we go away it's plenty of rest beforehand, a disabled room and transport everywhere.

But it's still a life. It's far from ideal, but I'm not going to let ME take away anything else. I'm a fighter and I'm not giving up.

Charlotte Cann

LIFE WITH *Sarah-Jayne*

The six months leading up to 14th September 2013 I was the happiest and fittest I had ever been. After recovering from the most severe and longest bout of depression I had ever experienced that started in January 2012 I had really turned my life around and had started to make exciting plans for the long term; life was good!

I had a busy social life and was very active with kayaking and weight training and I loved my job, which was managing a team of support workers who supported adults with learning difficulties.

Then, in September 2014, I went to Bulgaria as a volunteer for a charity and after two tough weeks I came back very tired, but it was to be expected after what I had just done. But what I didn't expect was to wake up two mornings later and not be able to get out of bed. I felt a level of exhaustion I had never experienced before. The year that followed was the most horrendous year of my life.

I was initially diagnosed with depression but while I accepted it, it didn't make sense because I was so happy leading up to this point. I had no reason for the depression to return. I now know that it wasn't depression but the start of ME. However, depression soon followed.

My physical symptoms fluctuated; some days I thought I was ok and getting better followed by days when the exhaustion would hit me hard and, over time, other symptoms started such as muscle aches, severe headaches and tender glands. I was suffering from cognitive issues that affected things such as loss of memory, my balance, and the ability to find the right words.

I had become a prisoner to my bedroom and some days to my bed where I had to spend most of my time alone because just being in the same room with someone else exhausted me even more. I started to suspect there was something more going on with me and I suggested to my GP on a few occasion that I thought I had ME, or as doctors prefer to call it, Chronic Fatigue Syndrome. My GP kept on dismissing this so I kept on pushing myself with exercising on the days when my symptoms weren't so severe, because that is what normally helps depression. But, unfortunately, all I was doing was making the invisible illness, ME, worse.

Eventually in May 2014 I saw a psychiatrist and begged her in floods of tears to let me have Electric Convulsive Therapy. Fortunately she said no and said that she suspected I may have Chronic Fatigue Syndrome and I knew then my suspicions had been correct all along. I started to treat the illness as ME and gradually, over the months, the depression improved, then in August 2014 I got the official diagnosis of ME.

The ME continued to be a roller coaster and, eventually, I had to leave my job, and I now face bankruptcy. I was told there is no cure for ME but people can learn to manage it. It's now the end of February 2015 and for the last couple of months I feel I am learning to manage it. I am able to do quite a bit more - no thanks to the NHS, but as a result of my reading about the condition and meeting other people online with the illness who have given me advice. I have been offered a place on a course through the NHS to learn about how to live with the condition, but I have not been well enough to attend it.

I now take a large amount of expensive supplements and eat a very healthy diet, which I can barely afford on the benefits I receive. I have learnt how to pace myself and I practice Mindfulness daily, which all contribute to a more bearable life but that is, unfortunately, still spent mainly in my bedroom on my own.

But it's not all doom and gloom; I have formed some great friendships through Facebook with other people who have ME and also Fibromyalgia that has similarities to ME and is just as much misunderstood and stigmatised.

There are many support groups on Facebook where we can both seek and offer support and advice. This prompted me to start my own Facebook group for people with ME and Fibromyalgia who live in Bristol, and I now have over eighty members and some of us have met for coffee through this group. One of the other positive things that has come about from being chronically ill is that it has changed me for the better as a person.

I have become more compassionate and patient towards others and I have an appreciation for the small things in life that I always took for granted, and I notice beauty in things that I had not noticed before. I hope one day with careful management and the supplements I will get some of my old life back, but I know there are no guarantees. And, if I do manage it, I know I am in for a long journey, but it's a journey that I'm not making alone now that I have many online friends for mutual support.

Sarah-Jayne

LIFE WITH *Sharon Klb*

I was travelling in 2006/2007 and was bitten by a tick in Kruger National Park on the last leg of my journey.

My daughter was sitting next to me, when I scratched the back of my neck and unfortunately removed the head of the tick. I became ill a few months after returning to the UK and I became very depressed too. This started to cause the breakup of my relationship and, when I finally went to see my GP, she sent tests for Lymes Disease, which came back inconclusive after too long....I then started to suffer lots of ME/CFS symptoms and she decided that it was probably a secondary condition.

My health has deteriorated greatly since then - changing my whole life. My present GP sent me for a re-test last year...the doctor then getting giddy at the fact he thought I had sleep apnoea! I need the expensive test, which is private, but I can't afford the fee.

Sharon Klb

LIFE WITH *Ema*

Myalgic Encephalomyelitis - Not easy to say, not easy to live with.

When I think of my story I know that I am luckier than many but not as lucky as some. This invisible chronic condition has plagued me over twenty-five years of my life, remaining invisibly undiagnosed but leaving a very visible mark on my daily life. However, for many years I was the only one aware of the scars.

It is hard to exactly pinpoint when I became aware that I didn't have the same tolerance and thresholds as other people but in my late teens, after a bout on glandular fever at sixteen, I found myself leaving parties early as I was too tired to stay up all night with my friends and if I did I would pay by falling ill a few days later. This pattern remained with me and is with me still.

Whenever my body reached a point where I became too fatigued I would have what I later came to call my 'black out days'. Visits to the doctor's in the early 90's yielded no answers and I just came to accept these 'black out days' as part of my existence. They didn't stop me gaining my degree or completing my PGCE in Drama Education but I appeared to find the rigours tougher than most, constantly feeling ill and poorly.

I qualified as a Teacher in 1993 and began what has been an amazing but completely exhausting career. Teaching IS exhausting, ask anyone in the profession and they will tell you the same. I just accepted that my tiredness and propensity to illness was due to the stresses of the job and the long and emotional hours I put in. Within six weeks of starting as an NQT I became quite poorly, the same symptoms which had sporadically made themselves apparent in the previous years - swollen glands, a searing pain in my head that made my eyes cave in and go black, the ability to sleep for almost forty eight hours without waking, wobbly legs, and the feeling that I had a terrible case of flu.

A trip back to the Dr and I was offered Prozac, as the Dr believed that I was suffering from stress, and the symptoms I was experiencing were just a result of finding the rigours of being a NQT stressful. Naive and willing to accept this diagnosis I started to take the medication. Granted I felt less anxious but the symptoms did not disappear. I came off the drugs nine months later as I was still having my 'black out days'. Then my body decided to take matters into its own hands and within a four year span I had my gallbladder, appendix, and tonsils out - each time returning to work within four weeks, sometimes less. Did I ever give my body time to recover? Who knows?

My illness record was not great and pressure was put on me by my then Head - a very unsympathetic and hard woman - who said to my mother when she rang to say I was in hospital after the emergency appendectomy 'When is she coming back to work, she is letting the students down by being away so often'.

Every day I was ill, I felt guilt, which is still with me to this very day and in many ways has contributed to my anxiety over always being ill, and this incident was some sixteen years ago.

Determined to deal with my issues I tried homeopathy, juice cleanses, herbal medicine, raw food diets, you name it, I have, in the last twenty-five years, tried it, and whilst there was sometimes an alleviation in symptoms my same old 'black out days' would haunt me every half term. In the twenty-one years I have been teaching I have only had one half term, yes one half term, when I have not had a day off with a 'black out day or days'. That does not make a good attendance record. Yet my passion for my job and my willingness to go the extra mile for my students when I was well meant that I NEVER let the students down and they have always excelled in their exams.

I have to say this, as I have to acknowledge that despite having been plagued by this illness all this time I have always put my students first, very often ahead of myself. When times have been tough I would come home and go to bed at 7pm just so I could be back in school the following day. School productions became an utter nightmare for me, as I would always 'crash due to the long hours and after each production I would be struck down with a major infection.

Colleagues have tolerated me but I know that they have been resentful of the days I have off seeing me as a 'malingerer' no matter what I do when I am there. This has been a constant source of stress and upset for me. Why was I always ill when nobody else was? Why did my body just give up on me? Why, when I was ill, could I not struggle in like everyone else? What was wrong with me? But no amount of blood tests gave any answers.

This pattern never fluctuating but was very much part of my life. My husband, whom I married in 2006, just accepts that he did not marry a party animal. In 2008 our son arrived in a flurry of drama on Friday 13th June by emergency caesarean section and was a SCBU baby for the first four weeks of his life. Ironically, whilst I was on maternity leave with a quite sick baby my symptoms were not as exacerbated as they had been. I would surmise now that this was down to the fact that I was sleeping when the baby slept and was getting more rest than when I was working.

When my son was nine months old I returned to work four days a week, and in the last four years my symptoms have been more pronounced than ever. It seems obvious to me now that I have been diagnosed with ME: More physical stress, more emotional stress, less time to stop and rest.

I hate to think about the time I have lost with my son due to my 'black out days' and the fact that I did not have any further children because I just knew I couldn't cope physically with another child, and having to work makes me sad but I am so grateful that I have him.

This illness that has been with me (which up until recently didn't have a name) has taken so much from me, and robs so much from so many, and it is only now that I have a diagnosis that I have sympathy and understanding from my colleagues. After twenty- five years things got so bad with my anxiety over being ill that last year I began to have major panic attacks and hideous bouts of insomnia, which meant that every day was a 'black out day'. I was forced to have a week off work and go back onto Prozac after twenty years. I decided to keep a diary charting my 'ill days' as well as to take up running. Exercise had become quite important to me in the last eighteen months but I would always suffer with exhaustion after a heavy workout. In July 2014 I ran my first (and it now looks like last) 10K for Great Ormond Street Hospital. I finished the race in a not so fast one hour and twelve minutes, and came home and slept for two solid hours. Was it the training and running that bought me to where I am now or the stress of a job which has become more difficult? I don't know.

But September 2014 marked a very dramatic downturn in my health. My 'black out days' were almost every day and I was finding it increasingly difficult to get up to go to work. My face was grey, my eyes caved in and sunken and my exhaustion level immense. I struggled through the days and most nights fell asleep with my son on his bed at 7pm. I became irritable, emotional and utterly fed up with things so I went back to the Dr and demanded to be referred onwards. It was these blood tests, which showed irregularities, that meant my referral was fast tracked and on December 10th I had an appointment at the Clinical Immunology department at The Royal Free Hospital in London.

After describing my symptoms the consultant turned to me and said 'You have a classic case of ME which you already know'. Did I know? Yes, No, I don't know. I wasn't as sick as other people, I was mobile, and I had a career... I wasn't like people I had read about with ME, but how much did I really know about the illness? It wasn't until after my diagnosis that I started to read up on it and there it was in black and white: My life for the last twenty-five years. Yes, I have had a life and a career but it has been TOUGH TOUGH

TOUGH and I never really knew why until December.

My body had crashed into relapse and over the last four months I have experienced a prolonged period of poor health. For once I have actually stopped work and gone on sick leave, I finally have the diagnosis which means I can give my body the rest it clearly needs. My days at the moment are very calm. I am sleeping late and doing very little during the day, but make it a priority to go and collect my son from school at 3.30pm, something I have not had the pleasure of doing regularly as I have always been at school myself. I am charting each day for my symptoms and each day at the moment is different, some good, some bad, some still 'black', but I know what I am dealing with.

I don't know how long I will be off work but for once I am putting myself first and finding out what my limits are. I know that this is a condition for life but I do not want it to be what defines me, it has defined and shaped every section of my life for twenty-five years, the parties I have missed, the outings, the theatre trips, the things I haven't done just so that I don't get to tired and become ill for work. The last few months have taught me a great deal; that I am lucky in many ways that my ME has at least allowed me to lead a life but perhaps most importantly I don't have to feel guilty or bad or apologetic about being ill.

LIFE WITH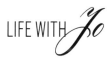

I first fell ill in 2001 at the age of sixteen. I had a nasty bout of tonsillitis that antibiotics wouldn't shift and some nasty stress in my personal life (which I won't go into).

After 6 months of not doing much other than staying in bed I was sent to see a specialist in Tilbury. He gave me the diagnosis of Chronic Fatigue Syndrome/Myalgic Encephalomyelitis.

By this point I had been thrown out of college due to my not being able to attend and didn't have any structure in my life (unless you count watching Neighbours).

I was advised to create a routine, and do everything in fifteen minute chunks. For example I could read a book for fifteen minutes, but then my next activity could not be a mental one (TV, computer, etc.).

I followed the rules as best I could, bearing in mind I was a teenager! I built on what I could do slowly and by the time I was twenty-one I would say I was fully well and in my mind would never be ill again! I lived a normal life for the next seven years. I worked, I passed my motorcycle riding test and enjoyed a few summers of riding. I got married, had two kids, re located and then bam...........!

In the early months of 2013 I was very stressed, I suffered a chest infection followed by an ear infection and just didn't pick up.

My GP said that it was post viral fatigue and I would improve after a few weeks. My mum said it could be my ME coming back and I should start following the rules again. I should have listened to my mum! It took me the best part of six months to come to terms with the idea that it was the ME back. I had to stop driving due to the dizziness and fatigue that had taken over my life.

We moved back to Whitstable in the October of 2013, which very much helped with the reduction of stress!

When we moved back the idea of having to get my eldest to and from school was scary. I knew I needed to take my youngest to toddler groups, which was daunting, and going into town to run errands was out of the question.

Now, seven months on, I can manage the school run without becoming a tearful wreck by Friday. I can go to the odd toddler group, although I do struggle with these due to the over stimulation, noise, people, heat. And amazingly I can even get into town using my electric tricycle and run errands!

I am amazed with how far I have come, and I hope I will continue to improve and perhaps next time notice the warning signs.

LIFE WITH *Julie Holliday*

I first got ill about eighteen years ago at the age of twenty-nine. Although perhaps it really started a year earlier when I took more than a month to get over a virus and was diagnosed with post viral fatigue. At the time I thought I was at the peak of my health. I had an active and demanding job as a Residential Social Worker, which I loved, and I volunteered at a youth counselling agency. I was extremely fit: I did yoga every day and either swam, ran, or did aerobics about five times a week. I also had a great social life but I didn't sleep much!

One day I felt that I was coming down with a virus. I rested up but it never fully materialized. However, as soon as I tried to work I was hit with extreme exhaustion and pain that nobody could explain. My response was to push; I was determined to get better. But instead I just got worse and could barely look after myself.

I was lucky to get a diagnosis of ME within about three months. At least it meant I could read up about what little was known about it. But I was frustrated that all my doctor wanted to do was to treat me with antidepressants. Eventually we agreed on a low dose of amitriptyline, which helped me sleep better and eased the pain and tension in my muscles a little. Then I started a T'ai chi class and started seeing an acupuncturist with slow but positive results. After six months I started back to work a few hours at a time. After another six months I was working half time but I knew that even though I was doing a lot better, it wasn't good for me to work when I was having a bad day, and there was no predicting my bad days when the work rota was drawn up!

By then I had accepted that I had a chronic illness and resolved not to put my life on hold until I was better. I knew I just needed to learn how to live it in a different way to keep within my energy limits. So I decided to leave work and go travelling again and headed off around South America. So what! If I couldn't walk the Inca trail - I could still visit Machu Picchu! So what! If I couldn't carry my backpack - I could get a taxi from the bus station to the hostel! The best thing about travelling was that I was wonderfully free to respond to how I was feeling on each day. I could do nothing on my bad days and it was very easy to pace! I had a wonderful time and little by little my health improved.

By the time I returned to England I had improved enough to live a relatively normal life, all be it a sedentary one. I was still unable to increase my physical activity without post-exertional malaise. I then decided to build on my Psychology Degree and take an Advanced Diploma in person centered counselling. It was something I knew from my voluntary work that I was good at but had always resisted because I couldn't imagine a job that involved sitting down all day! Now it fits much better with the way ME/CFS dictated that I live my life.

Gradually my health continued to improve as I continued practising a way of being that I'd been learning through my interest in Taoist philosophy. This involved accepting my daily limitations and minimising both mental and physical exertion. I became an expert at relaxed effortlessness.

5 years after ME/CFS first hit me, I found myself looking down from the peak of a mountain (Helvellyn) I'd hiked up, feeling like a blind woman who had regained her sight. I knew I was well again, I had beaten this illness. Unfortunately that's not the end of my story.....

With my full health returned my itchy feet could no longer be ignored. For the next few years I traveled and chose work that enabled me to live for today. Instead of taking care of people I had fun: I did six ski seasons in the Sierra Nevada Mountains in Spain, first as a Rep and a Ski Guide and later as a Ski Instructor. In the summers I worked as a Walking Guide, Group Tour Leader and Hotel Receptionist. In between seasons I picked cherries, I temped, I 'wwoofed' and did whatever I had to, to get by. And I experienced joy on a daily basis.

Then, after a relatively stressful ski season with money worries and a nightmare flat mate, I picked up a virus on a plane journey. I was on my way to a brief, between-season visit to family and friends. I had so little time to catch up with everybody that against my better judgement, I ignored my body's need for rest and rushed around seeing everyone as planned. My first day back in Spain (after seven years of full health) I was horrified to realise I had those familiar symptoms again. Determined to look on the bright side I thought that if I rested and put all my previous learning back into action, it might just end up being a short term post viral fatigue. My management kept my symptoms mild but a couple of months later I suffered a nasty tooth infection requiring two courses of antibiotics, and that was the start of a new complication.

My gut flora were thrown out of balance by the antibiotics and I developed intolerance to sugar. This gradually extended to wheat and gluten, then to yeast, vinegar and mushrooms. Now I had a new challenge to deal with, (one

I still haven't overcome completely).

Unable to do another ski season, my job as a hotel receptionist was extended to ten months a year. It was an easy, sedentary job that I was familiar with and I could live a relatively stress free life in a very beautiful village surrounded by supportive friends. Three years later, after learning to meditate at a yoga retreat, I suddenly knew that I wasn't giving my health enough of a chance working all the hours that I did. It also became clear to me that I needed to share all I'd learned about self-help. I made the decision to leave Spain and return to my parents' house in England in order to write my book. I started blogging as the ME/CFS Self-Help Guru and later decided to qualify as a life coach. Living at my parents I was able to support myself with part time work at the local convenience store.

I'm now very excited to be running my own business as a holistic life coach with the aim of helping others manage chronic illness better, make their contribution and live their dream. I may not be completely recovered again yet but I'm well on the way to living my dream!

www.mecfsselfhelpguru.com

Julie Holliday
(The ME/CFS Self-Help Guru)

LIFE WITH *M Harding*

Ok, I was never destined to become Jessica Ennis. What am I talking about? She wasn't even born when I was. Anyway, I guess what I'm trying to say is that although I would never have been an Olympian, I considered myself to be relatively fit. Hockey, basketball, taekwondo, badminton and a three-mile run every morning training to run the mile for the school in the county trials! I have always worked from... well as soon as I could really.

I had glandular fever in the year that I did my A levels – sigh, but I did them and failed so redid them again and passed them so you could say I was a fighter! It seems that glandular fever is quite common in the ME community!

After that came my first 'real' jobs! I temped for a while, working as a personal assistant at an aerospace company, which I loved, and doing various other jobs that did not seem as glamorous or important but money makes the world go round so they say! Thereafter I served twelve years in the Court Service in various courts in various places, departments and roles! I was married to my amazing husband and we moved to London. Two wonderful children later, a son and daughter, we found ourselves in Dover.

After I had my children, unfortunately, I had an ectopic pregnancy which led to depression and so I took early retirement. I thought 1996 was our annus horribilis – Ha! What did I know! Anyway, again I found myself fighting back to life with the help of various therapists. (Cheryl Cole had nothing on me!).

In 1999 my daughter started school and I volunteered at the local volunteer bureau and became an Akela (Cub leader) to fill my life which had suddenly become much more peaceful - I don't know why that might have been!!! I also helped out at the children's school listening to children read and helping with painting and crafts. The Head teacher offered me a Teaching Assistant job teaching children to read but also helping children who had behavioural needs. I loved it and it was a novelty to be paid for something I really enjoyed!

I had a sudden urge to possess a degree, Lord knows why, in fact he probably does! I went part-time and studied for a BSc in Psychology with Early Childhood Studies (ECS) for six years and although it required dedication and a heap of hard work I got my degree!

I went back to work full time and the ECS element in particular informed my job. So there I was running an after-school gardening club, a self-portrait club and helping the head at table tennis club. Happy times!

Now, I am asthmatic and so I take everything medical offered to me; flu jabs, pneumonia jabs etc. Every year I get a chest infection since I had my tonsils removed twenty years ago, and 2014 was no exception. This was a bad dose though and led to me having bed rest rather than hospital. I returned to work not feeling very special and within a week I was off work again, in bed feeling very ill and sorry for myself. I saw several doctors but by the time I saw my own GP I was in a bad way and had to write down all my symptoms as my memory was basically shot away. He was the first person to explain the dreadful illness I had: I was diagnosed with post-viral fatigue syndrome.

He referred me for Cognitive Behavioural Therapy (CBT) and gave me anti-depressants. Well to quote another song 'the drugs don't work' so he changed them to fluoxetine. In the weeks before the new drug did eventually work, it felt like a long time!! I felt lower than I had ever been in my life; I was given a crisis number 'in case', in short, I was suicidal. My amazing husband and daughter were caring for me, the second time for my husband. I am so lucky!

Now this all sounds very doom and gloom and, indeed, this was a very dark period in my life and I still have dark moments nearly one year on. The wretched illness has changed my life dramatically, I couldn't work and struggled to walk a mile, and so my usual twenty mile walks at the weekend were out of the question. But what has this taught me? It has taught me to value small moments, to make my ambitions realistic, celebrate my achievements and not beat myself up when I cannot get out of bed. 'Isn't it ironic', Alanis Morissette sang, well she didn't quite understand the meaning of the word, but it is ironic that ME/CFS causes you to sleep so much but that sleep is not satisfying or healing. People just don't comprehend the difference between tiredness and fatigue which consumes your very being!

I still have weekly CBT and this has taught me coping strategies such as progressive muscle relaxation and Mindfulness, both of which really help if I have the energy to do them every day.

Coping with M.E/CFS is hard work, make no bones about it: you do have to make an effort to survive it! Some things you can work through but there are also 'those days' that you have to tolerate along with the good days or hours when, for example, you leave the house or even your bed! At the start when you are feeling so vulnerable and scared, the Facebook forums and books are a must so that you can be informed about the illness. Choose with care though! Ask someone with ME. Friends and family do eventually 'get it'. I'm sure I'm not the only one who has fallen asleep on the phone to the mother only to wake with a jump when she called my name!!

So my coping strategies....... Surround yourself with positivity in everything and build a support network, not out of bricks, but people, family, friends and medical practitioners. If they're not positive get different ones! Be compassionate to yourself, you are ill! Do a Sudoku every day or something similar to challenge those little grey cells which, believe it or not, are still there, they just need prodding more than they used to! (Ha! who am I kidding sometimes they need a defibrillator!). Take vitamins as recommended by a practitioner such as Dr Sarah Myhill.

Use this as a learning/teaching experience: no-one fully understands this illness until they 'get it' and in my experience it is different for each individual. Learn about yourself and teach other people! You can survive this!

LIFE WITH *Gem P*

Life never goes the way you plan. I, for one, did not expect to be diagnosed with a chronic illness aged thirteen.

I was in year nine of secondary school and was looking forward to starting my GCSEs. I had a good group of friends and social life; I was a normal teenager… Until I started to notice things – I was always tired when I got home from school. I had headaches daily and my legs started to ache after a short walk. I put it off as hormones, normal teenage stuff, until my school break. The whole six weeks were spent in the comforts of my bed. I was too tired to get up or get dressed. I went to the doctors, concerned about how I was feeling. They ran a never ending series of blood tests, testing for everything possible. But everything was normal.

That's when I was told I had Myalgic Encephalomyelitis. I was shocked, I couldn't believe it.

I returned to school, tried to pretend things were normal. But then I started to struggle, my attendance dropped and my social life wavered. I ended up dropping some of my GCSE subjects and doing half days at school, which were eventually cut down to nothing.

My school friends turned on me, accusing me of being lazy and that I was making it up. I cried myself to sleep every night. Why would I make it up? Who would choose to live a life exhausted? I started to get bullied online; horrible things were said about me. About my 'so called' illness.

I was then diagnosed with depression and anxiety. Although I was going through a bad time, I had my partner to support me. He was my rock. My last light, my hope. He moved into my parent's house to look after me and I can't fault him. The last year of school went by like a flash; I forgot school and everyone in it.

Until prom, I had always dreamt of going to the prom, wearing a beautiful dress and feeling like a princess, just for one night. But I wasn't allowed to go; the school said my attendance was too low. Seeing the photos of my old friends, smiling at the camera, looking beautiful, it hurt.

I then realised what I had lost. What I can never get back. Time went by and I stayed the same – my illness held me back so much, but I learnt to cope with it. But then I started to feel better. I had more energy; I could move my muscles without severe pain… I was overwhelmed with happiness. I thought I was cured! But of course, I was only in remission and a relapse was shortly around the corner.

I relapsed when I was sixteen years old. I was devastated to find that I was more poorly than before. I was now completely housebound and mostly bedbound. My partner was still by my side, helping me as much as he could. I shortly moved out; our family life was stressful and impacting on my health. But sadly, due to unforeseen circumstances, my fiancé and I had to move back to my hometown, although we found a place of our own.

Shortly after moving back, I started to feel very unwell – getting severe pain in my ears that would make me scream. I found out that I had a severe ear infection that was very close to spreading into my blood. I was very unwell and placed on antibiotics for six weeks. The pain and exhaustion I felt during that time isn't something I would wish on anyone.

My health rapidly got worse after finally killing the infection. Every day was full of pain and exhaustion. I didn't see any sort of future for myself and feel into a deep depression. It was then I was also diagnosed with Fibromyalgia.

Fast forward to now, I am still struggling massively with my physical and mental health. Every day is a struggle, and I now need crutches to walk.

I wish I could be a normal eighteen year old: Work, university, going out! But I know that isn't possible. I am so glad to have my fiancé by my side, he does everything to help me, and I know I am so lucky because some people will never find someone like that. My social life has also picked up; a few friends from my school days have now reconnected and visit me, and expressed how sorry they were for treating me like they did. I know my life is never going to be how I planned it to be. I will miss out on so much. But this is the life I was given, so I have to make the best of it.

LIFE WITH *Bill Clayton*

M.E. and ME

I ran, I swam, it's who I am
I laughed, had fun, enjoyed the sun.
I was doing such when this begun.

Felt a chill on a good warm day
Aches and pains that won't go away
Like the flu, I heard it said
But arms and legs are made of lead.

Can't remember what I was about to say
Simple words have gone astray
Can't make a choice between two simple things
Someone else is pulling my strings.

I try to read, but it only drains
Focusing harder, just scrambles my brains
The dark clouds descend, lead to despair
The weight of three men sinks into my chair

No outward sign to give a clue
No bandage, mark, no black and blue
Strange, it seems I always look well
Look from this side, then you could tell
Remove the mask for a day to see
The evil face of this beast called M.E.
Like a thief in the night it takes away
Your hope, your strength, your friends
Your likes, your loves your chance to play
And never makes amends

All we want is to be believed
And trusted when we say
Hey GP, can't you see
We didn't ask to be this way
This is real, a real big deal
As big as the 'popular' ills
It needs to be taught, given some thought
Not just a bundle of pills

We don't have a choice, we need a real voice
Give us some hope TODAY
So don't be doubting, we're gonna keep shouting
We're just not going away.

Bill Clayton

LIFE WITH *Anon*

I want to explain as much as possible about my life with ME and the devastating impact it has had both on me and my family.

My life has been a nightmare for the past nineteen years since I contracted this disease. Every day there is a new obstacle; it is one long uphill struggle. I was an active and creative person before I was struck down overnight with flu-like illness. I even moved to Norfolk largely because I am keen on conservation, and I love walking in the countryside so much. I particularly enjoy horse riding, walking on the beach, dancing and I really don't like to sit still. For a holiday, I chose to go to places like Scotland, Ireland, Wales - although I have not had a holiday for at least thirteen years now.

I am a qualified dental nurse, I enjoy hard work, loved my job, and I like to earn the respect of others through my actions.

My experience with ME, right from day one, has been that the majority of people did not believe I was sick, most especially my ex-husband. It has been absolute hell starting from the first visit to a doctor - who told me to take vigorous exercise daily and lied on my medical notes about the purpose of my visit; I went for flu but instead she wrote that I went for depression! I followed her advice and carried on forcing myself to carry on with the vigorous exercise, and as a result I became completely bedridden for the next two years.

I don't know how I have endured it, except that I have no choice, because, in addition to the pain and other horrible symptoms, I believe it is largely because of my ex-husband's disbelief in my illness that my marriage broke down. In any case, from day one I was left to rot in bed for the better part of two years, and my daughter's childhood was ruined because her father kept out of the way, and left her to be my sole carer when she was only nine or ten years old.

I have tried time and time again to go back to work, but I have not been able to keep working because of physical illness and cognitive difficulties, and I have had to put my longed-for Art degree on permanent hold because of the same. I have lost count of the endless number of regular negative experiences and hardships I have endured over the last nineteen years as a result of other people's negative attitude to ME.

The consensus seems to be that ME sufferers are just liars and malingerers. Although I cannot possibly imagine what reason anyone thinks I might want to be like this, or what such people might imagine I could have possibly gained, because it has been nothing but loss and grief from the start. Perhaps people think that I must like having my reputation, my credibility and my whole life ruined by a painful and debilitating illness that nobody believes in, and I must think it's fun to be isolated, broke and housebound; when all the time I have ample courage, endurance, qualifications, intelligence, experience and talent - enough to enjoy a full life and a very good living - if only I wasn't ill with ME.

I eventually achieved a remission somewhere along the line but, stupidly, thought I was cured. After I had to take an intermission from my BA hons Art course because of a relapse, I still continued working for another year as a breakfast waitress. During that time, I was unable to take time off when I was sick, because if I did, I would never have been at work at all. I used to take a handful of painkillers in the morning and drag myself into work no matter what. I hid my illness from the people that I worked with because I was ashamed, and I was really stressed out and paranoid that they would find out that I was ill. I was much too sick for any socializing or housework, for a year my home was filthy, but all I could do after work was go to bed.

It was at this time that I went to see a counsellor because I had started drinking and it scared me. To cut a long story short he told me that I was in denial about my illness, and I had to work on accepting it, and telling people about it.

I am a responsible person and, before I was finally forced to give up work, I had a current account that was always in credit, a good work record, a steady income, and a very healthy bank savings account. When I was finally forced to give up work due to my second relapse, I suddenly had no income, so I went to the Community Legal Service for their help with making applications for the right benefits. At the time I was often bedridden, virtually housebound and always made worse by any activities.

Unfortunately, I was wrongly advised by, my then, CLS representative to apply for Income Support. I wonder why she did this because it seems like a basic thing to me. When I had finally managed to send in my income support application, I was eventually told - after perhaps two further months or so of waiting - that I had been wrongly advised because I should have been told to apply for Incapacity Benefit. My award then had to be given from the later date of my second application for Incapacity Benefit, rather than my earlier application for Income Support. In the end, I believe it was fully six months before I received my first payment of Incapacity Benefit from the DWP.

I believe it was a further eighteen months before I received any help from Income Support towards paying my mortgage, the money for which payments I had been taking out of my meager incapacity benefit so I did not get behind with them. It was not until years later that I was finally advised to apply for Disability Living Allowance by the CLS. I asked a CLS representative to help me complete the application forms because of my cognitive difficulties, and I believe it was because of my cognitive difficulties and communication problems, and her own personal skepticism about ME that the CLS representative filled out my application form incorrectly, putting her own beliefs in some places instead of asking me to answer the questions, and as a result of her mistakes I was not awarded the Mobility DLA that I was actually entitled to.

I made a formal complaint, but to no avail. I also contacted my local Disability Rights Service who told me that the CLS representative who made this mistake was in fact breaking the law, because I had told her I had cognitive difficulties; so when I was tired, instead of guessing the answers, she should have stopped the interview when I became mentally exhausted, and rescheduled it for another day. She definitely should not have asked me to sign the forms as she did without getting me to read them first. Even so, they thought that I stood no chance at all of proving that my CLS representative had acted improperly. Further, I was warned that if I contested the actions of the CLS representative I would be put through an awful lot of stress and upset, and they would still win.

When I wrote to that CLS representative, she told me that I was lucky to get DLA at all with my controversial illness, and if I attempted to get an increase in my DLA award, then I stood to risk losing it completely. So, because I am always paranoid, because in my experience nobody believes that ME is a real physical illness, it was not difficult to scare me off. It was not until years later that I aggressively pursued this application and received my full DLA Mobility award, but this could not be backdated to the date of my earlier application.

Meanwhile, I was so sick that until I was referred to the Social Services, I had to pay out of my own pocket for the practical help I needed at home, and I had a mortgage to pay, a home to run and a child to support, and very little income.

Since Dr. Terry Mitchell had advised me to be a lot stricter in my activity management when I saw him in 2004, I found these enforced restrictions completely intolerable, and I found that I really couldn't stick to a proper pacing routine at all. Whatever I do I still manage to stubbornly refuse to give in until I have made myself ill.

He had carefully explained that my previous 'boom and bust' pattern of coping with the illness, and my tendency to push my limitations, had made matters much worse, especially in regard to the cognitive difficulties and the resulting deterioration of my draughtsmanship skills; and he advised me that if I were to manage my activities much more carefully, and avoid overdoing things, it was his firm belief that my cognitive faculties would improve.

I enjoy working and being efficient, I like the social side of work and I enjoy helping people and meeting people in a work environment, and I had been a very efficient, fully qualified Dental Nurse for many years. But my cognitive difficulties alone made it impossible for me to work, and I am so often stuck in bed. But because my work as a painter was so important to me, (having been forced in December 2002 to take another temporary intermission from my B.A. Fine Art studies at Anglia Ruskin), after years of enforced inactivity and social isolation, determined to make the best of this unbearable situation, I thought that if I were to use a power wheelchair, I would be able to stick to my activity management and avoid boom and bust, while at the same time still get out of the house a lot more. I would at least be able to take my dog for a walk, and I especially hoped I would be enabled to return to university on a part time basis, particularly since I already had enough credits towards the course from my HND Fine Art qualification in order to start in the second year. So even on a part time basis I could have completed my BA in four years.

I did not discuss this with my new GP, Dr H, because, although by that time she had visited Dr. Mitchell at Great Yarmouth and professed that she had a good understanding of ME, I did not really trust her. I often found her to be extremely odd, often making completely inexplicable remarks or laughing at the most inappropriate moments during our consultations; often grinning from ear to ear when she was telling me very bad news indeed.

I was also aware by that time, that my GP was living in the house next door to my ex-husband and his new wife (who had been my 'best friend' for around ten years until I became bedridden with ME, when she and my husband started an affair).

When Dr. H first diagnosed my illness, she began by saying she 'knew nothing' about ME and I was very impressed by this apparent honesty. She then went to visit Dr. Terry Mitchell at his clinic and apparently became a firm advocate for Dr. Mitchell's beliefs that ME is a purely physical illness.

I often expressed my fears to Dr H that my illness might not be real, or that nobody believed in it. I knew that my ex-husband thought I was simply mad, and that just about everybody assumed that ME was some form of depression, but each time I had expressed my fears, Dr. H was always very quick to reassure me. Yet I now believe, that each time Dr. H wrote a referral note for me, she very carefully and deliberately 'primed' the person she referred me to so that they would think they already knew something extremely derogatory about me, before they even had a chance to meet me.

This is not the place to go into detail about all the events that took place in my private life but I am of the firm opinion that my ex-husband and his wife often undermined me, had a detrimental influence on my GP, who in turn failed to support me and, in fact, discredited me with the people she referred me to. Time and time again, after a referral note by Dr. H, I have been greeted with skepticism and often outright rudeness and open derision from professional people I have never met before. As a consequence, I am in no doubt that it was because of this I went from bad to worse.

At one point I, apparently, had a TIA or mini stroke. I suddenly couldn't speak (my family thought I was having a stroke). I had tried to talk to the emergency doctor on the telephone but I had great difficulty with word retrieval, which is an everyday experience for ME patients, so the emergency doctor had to talk to my Aunt instead, and I was writing notes to communicate with my aunt. He said that it 'seemed very bad' and told her to bring me in to A& E as soon as possible.

I learned later that the type of blood thickening drugs I was being given at that time were highly dangerous and should not be given to people who are immobilized as I was with ME - not even for long aeroplane flights. However, I believe that the hospital team implied that hypochondria or mental illness as the cause of this visit to A&E, a completed unfounded suggestion. I am convinced that the drugs Utovlan and Mefenamic Acid, which I had only ceased taking the day before the event, were very likely indeed to have been the cause. I made a complaint in the end because I felt I had to do something to prevent there being any ill effects from these unfortunate insinuations.

Once I had my power wheelchair I planned to return to my BA fine art studies but Dr H flatly refused to help me to apply for a disabled students allowance, which was necessary to physically enable me to complete the last two years of my BA fine Art degree course.

That was the story eight years ago. I am too exhausted to say much more. Of course I never did get back to university, and currently I am still deteriorating and have been housebound and almost entirely bedridden for roughly four years now.

I do however, have new GP at a different surgery, who visits me from time to time and is very respectful. But I am too ill to get out to a hospital for any of the tests he wants to arrange for me, or to a dental surgery for treatment of several broken teeth.

I have had a dietician visit me at home for my food intolerances and am currently in touch with a Specialist Occupational Therapist from the ME Centre via e-mail. When my GP wants bloods they send the district nurse, and that is the full extent of the NHS medical care I currently receive.

But at least no one laughs in my face or pretends I am crazy now, so there is that much to be thankful for.

Anon

LIFE WITH *Louise*

When I was a child I never got ill. Well, very rarely, and I'm talking maybe once every couple of years, I'd get a virus or a sickness bug that kept me off school, but I'd always bounce back after a couple of days and within a week I'd be back to the usual routines of after-school clubs, swimming club, dance, drama, music lessons - the list went on.

I had a very lovely, busy life, full of so much fun. I was particularly into performing arts, and at the end of my last year at school I got an amazing chance to have a lead role in 'A Chorus Line' at the theatre linked to my school. It was brilliant, and being able to go flat out for something that I loved doing was something that I look back on with very fond memories!

At the end of 2007, I got tonsillitis. I got on with life as I had before - life couldn't stop just because I was poorly. I knew I'd be better very soon. It was a stubborn virus though, and after a week on antibiotics it still hadn't gone. I found that I was getting exhausted very quickly, but it didn't bother me as it wasn't too bad and I knew that it was because I'd had a bit of a rough ride with my tonsillitis. Eventually, the tonsillitis shifted - the sore throat faded and I was able to swallow again without feeling like all my food and drink was running through razor blades. The exhaustion, however, just didn't go - it actually started getting more intense. It wasn't really stopping me from living my day-to-day life; it was just making things take three times as long.

What was strange though was the exhaustion itself. Rather than being tired, or even really completely knackered, I felt a completely new type of total lack of strength. I just felt like my entire body had been filled with heavy sandbags and just couldn't keep myself going, despite my best efforts. It's still really difficult to describe to a non-sufferer, even now.

I'd also find that if I did a lot in a day, the day after or even the day after that I would struggle to walk to the end of the road without my muscles feeling sore, achy and painful and my strength draining in no time at all. I eventually went to the doctors after a few months, but instead of being told what the problem was and given something to fix it, the doctor didn't have a clue what was going on. Over the next few months I had so many blood tests and scans,

I had to fill in questionnaires and keep diaries, but nobody could tell me that there was anything wrong. ME was mentioned, but never followed up on. So I decided that it was just me, a change in lifestyle or something. I got on with it, thinking that maybe I was just different to other people.

In 2010 I graduated from university and started a PGCE in Secondary English. I loved the idea of being a teacher and was so excited about my career ahead. I started off really well, but towards the end of my first placement I went home one Friday evening with a headache and ended up being taken to A&E that night and kept in hospital with suspected meningitis. Even though I didn't have it and went home, I was struggling more and more from that point on.

Shortly after starting my second placement the idea of ME was seriously raised, but everything had to be investigated very thoroughly first. So along came lots more blood tests, questionnaires, ECGs, scans and many more different tests. I was sent to a doctor who specialised in ME, but by the time I got my appointment I'd had to go part-time with my PGCE and was spending my days off in bed feeling very weak, sick, painful and dizzy when I sat up or tried to get out of bed and do things. I had to be pushed around in a wheelchair which was so soul destroying and so humiliating, especially if I saw people that I knew - so I stopped going out. I was spiralling into this awful world where I could keep myself together and pass as a healthy person to the kids at work - just, but outside of school I was a total wreck.

I was almost relieved when I was eventually diagnosed with ME, but when I found out that there was no cure my heart completely plummeted and the only reaction I could find was to cry. A lot. For days, I felt so angry, scared, confused and isolated, especially because I knew nobody else with ME. I felt that I had been so very badly let down by my body. So I desperately started ploughing through forums, trying to find someone who could promise me that it would soon disappear. I didn't find that person, but I did make some of my closest friends today who have taught me that it's OK to have all those feelings, and to remember that you are never alone.

After pushing my body so hard to get through my PGCE I qualified as a teacher, but at a cost. My body completely crashed. I fell into a complete hell where I was lying in bed every day with a scarf over my eyes to block out the light, being fed small amounts of custard and juice because swallowing was just too painful and exhausting. Every day was a battle to just survive, to get through another day bearing the pain. I began to seriously question the point of carrying on, but I knew that I had to - I had no other option. In all honestly, it hit me emotionally as well as physically. Inside I was crying out to tell someone how very frustrated I was feeling, but I really couldn't. It felt like some people were trying to look for a psychological cause to pin to my symptoms, possibly because nobody could physically see what my body was going through - and I knew any emotional issue I was having was as a result of my physical illness, not the cause of it.

So I didn't open up to anyone, not even my boyfriend. Then I ended up in hospital for weeks and was met with the most painful and hurtful experience of all. The doctors and nurses just didn't believe that I was really ill. I couldn't understand why at all because I wasn't putting it on for a second and did not want to be there under any circumstances. They would make me do things that were making me cry and be sick because of how painful and ill it made me feel, and then push even more. And if I told them I just couldn't, they told me that I just needed to put mind over matter, asking if I wanted to get better. One nurse even told me that my friends and boyfriend would only come and see me for so long. Every day was miserable, painful and full of desperation - desperation to get better, but also desperation for someone to believe that I was genuinely trying my hardest to be as well as I could and to play to their tune, but my body just wouldn't follow.

I was very lucky when I was discharged to have the most amazing physiotherapist and occupational therapist working with me at home, and with carers visiting three times a day I started making small steps. I was bed bound still for a few months after being discharged from hospital, and during this time I made myself a bucket list. There were things like go downstairs, go for a walk, go on holiday, get a job, and move out of my mum and dad's house. Top of the list though was something I'd always wanted to do - see the Northern Lights. Even writing it down was just ridiculous. Nobody was able to tell me when, or if, I'd get better, so mentally I'd prepared myself that I could potentially be in that state permanently. I couldn't see how I'd ever get myself standing and walking again, so I never even gave it a second thought that seeing the Northern Lights could really happen one day.

On Christmas Day 2011, I went downstairs for the first time since the end of October/ beginning of November that year, apart from one hospital appointment where I'd been carried downstairs and back up by the ambulance crew. It felt amazing. A few days afterwards, I took my first steps unaided. From there I went from strength to strength with a lot of support and the right combination of proper, helpful professional advice, a brilliant, well planned combination of medication and being allowed to say 'no' when it got too much. By May that year, convinced that I'd got through the worst of the ME forever and that it was full steam ahead from there onwards, I'd got my first job at a school to do my NQT year.

Again, like my PGCE year, I started off OK but really struggled. I was once again making myself poorly. I just got myself through it, thanks to some seriously wonderful support from a few people who believed in me totally, and knew how important getting through the year was to me. I passed, but it was a bittersweet achievement as I knew I wouldn't be able to hold down a full time teaching job with ME like I'd planned. That was the time when I really had to accept that I had ME and stop burying my head in the sand. It was a really stressful, painful time and I wanted to be healthy so much that I began to feel incredibly suffocated by the ME. I left my job, but it wasn't all bad news. Thanks to many hours of talking and encouragement by some very special friends I decided that one day I would take my teaching career down a new and more manageable path. I took some time out to recover from ill health, and since late 2013 I've been working as a Learning Mentor.

Although very daunting and hard at first, coming to terms with my ME and accepting that I have to manage it properly has become easier with the right support and love from a few completely wonderful people around me. It's not been a smooth road at all, but learning to pace myself properly, sticking to a gluten-free diet and having the loveliest friends I could ask for looking after me when I'm poorly has meant I've got myself to a really good level. I still have my bad days physically and emotionally, I still get days where I just want to scream 'why?' at the world and desperately want the ME to just go, but overall I've got a fantastic life now and the ME has in many ways brought a lot of positives.

I still have physical boundaries, and if I want to do something it has to be very carefully planned well in advance so that I have chance to build up strength and recover afterwards.

I have a board in my kitchen where I plan out my whole week to make sure that every day I'm staying within my limits, and things have to become prioritised. During the working week especially, non-essential things are usually cut completely. I can't really be spontaneous like I used to and that can be very frustrating at times, but planning and managing my illness like that means that sometimes I can do things that I enjoy - especially seeing friends, I love doing that more than anything!

I'm not living a life that many people in their 20's would be living, but it works for me and I feel stronger now than I have done since the ME came along.

I've got a really lovely friend who has just been a complete rock and is a very special friend to me, and this February, she and I went to Norway. We went on a Northern Lights chasing trip and I met that biggest, most important but most unrealistic challenge on my wish list. I lay in the snow and felt so overwhelmed; it was so incredibly emotional, that I could only really acknowledge that I was the most proud I'd ever been. We even saw shooting stars - you can probably guess what I wished for! I don't think I'll ever find the words to describe what that night meant - I don't actually think there are any words. And that's coming from an English teacher!

Everything has taught me that miracles don't always come easily or often but they do happen. Even at your worst points there are always positives to take, and you just have to hang on to hope so much that the bad times will pass. I am so hopeful that they will find a cure for ME, but I have learnt that in the meantime it is really important to have dreams, however small, and make the effort to put your precious energy into doing things for YOU. Of course it's important to listen so carefully to your body and not go over your limits, but you need to think of yourself too.

Sometimes you have to think about your priorities - sometimes a phone call to a friend is more important than a clean bedroom for example. Life is so short, you can't just sit there and wait for good things to happen to you - you have to find them. And trust me; they will happen eventually, no matter tough it gets!

Louise

LIFE WITH *T.B*

I have been thinking of how to write this article, and I have come to the conclusion that it's going to end up as something like Louise's piece. I can only say how I have managed being ill and living alone as a single person. So, here it goes!

It started in 2002, and this is where the story begins.

Three years ago, in September 1998, I had a viral infection. At the time I was working full time for an insurance company. My job was telephone-based dealing with car accident claims. It was also on a shift pattern working between the hours of 8am and 8pm so some weeks I would be working 8am-4pm others 12pm-8pm or anything in between. After being ill I went back to work but never felt properly recovered. I was always tired, felt ill and had lots of strange symptoms. One day I'd have a sore throat so I'd go to bed early, next day I would be fine. This carried on until May 1999 when I had my thirtieth birthday. I had been on holiday in a caravan and found I couldn't do the things I would normally have done. I couldn't shop in the morning and go walking in the afternoon; I couldn't drive round all day looking at the countryside… In fact I felt awful.

I found myself sitting in my car in a car park crying my heart out for no reason. So I decided when I got home I would go to the doctor. I was then diagnosed with glandular fever, which was a relief as by then I'd decided I was going mad, and if life was always going to be like this I didn't want to continue. Living alone made life both easier and harder! I live in a flat with my cat Mogs, who was a rescue cat with strange attitudes and ideas!

When I was told I had glandular fever I was given a sick note for six weeks so I went home and slept, and slept, and slept. Mogs wasn't happy with this as she used to be shut out of the bedroom and would wake me up in the morning yowling and scratching the door. We soon came to an arrangement where I would leave the door open so if she got worried about me she could come in. That meant that most mornings I woke up to find a cat sitting on the bed quite happily watching me, which was a much better arrangement.

At first I would get up, feed Mogs, have breakfast and go back to bed. Get up have dinner and go back to bed. Get up have tea, feed Mogs and go back to bed. Not a very busy life, but it was all I could do.

This continued for a while so I had to force myself to do things like food shopping. I would go to the supermarket and walk around slowly leaning on my trolley and wondering what the staff would do if I passed out. I would get home feeling terrible and then have to get my shopping to the flat. Luckily the lifts are always working in our block unless there has been a major problem, which is very rare. After getting my shopping in I would go and put my car in the compound knowing I wasn't going out again that day and that if I didn't do it immediately I would forget to do it. That had happened to me before and I'd panicked thinking my car had been stolen, as it wasn't where it should be. I came out of the front door of the flats and there was my car. I never leave it outside as it's not safe but feeling ill I'd done just that.

After my six weeks off I went back to work deciding I was better now. My doctor had referred me to the local hospital to see a consultant in infectious diseases so I was going there every couple of weeks for blood tests. I didn't really know why at that point but quite honestly didn't care. I was told my glandular fever antibodies were off the scale and had tests to check my immune system. I was diagnosed as having Post Viral Chronic Fatigue secondary to glandular fever, which seemed a fair description of how I was feeling.

At work things were getting harder. I went to my Manager and told her of my illness and explained Id been advised to do no overtime. The company expects everyone to do at least fifteen hours overtime a month and I just couldn't do it. I got a letter from the hospital and the company agreed I needn't do the overtime. After a few weeks like this I found I just couldn't cope at all. I would be dealing with people on the phone who had been in car accidents and were much shaken and I would find myself being irritable or even crying with them. One day I just couldn't stop crying and couldn't explain why I was crying as I didn't feel unhappy just very ill. I was sent home and haven't been back since.

At home I was back to resting, sleeping and doing very little. My flat was looking a mess, very dusty and full of cat hairs. Food was a frozen meal from the supermarket as that was all I could cook. It went in the microwave or the oven and I could sit down until it was ready. If I didn't I was too tired to eat. Washing up happened when I ran out of cutlery or cups as the frozen meals were eaten from the carton and thrown away. If I had a day where I felt well I would clean the flat, move furniture and generally do way too much and make myself ill again.

Now I'm still off work but I have got into a routine which seems to suit me. I am feeling a lot better most of the time and only have occasional bad days.

My flat is still rather messy but now I can make sure the kitchen is clean and washing up is done.

I go to the supermarket but now I know that when I get home I can still do things which don't need much energy. I don't need to sleep all the time now but still have occasional afternoon snoozes when I feel tired! I still don't always do everything I feel I should within my flat.

I'll find that changing the bed can wear me out for the day, hoovering makes me ache and general cleaning can be left until I feel up to it.

I now have two cats after gaining Amber in November 1999 when she was a stray who was picked up by someone who couldn't keep her. That was a very stressful time as Mogs didn't appreciate the company and Amber turned out to be pregnant and had to be spayed very quickly. I just couldn't cope with kittens as well! The cats get on well now and keep each other amused when I'm not up to much. They also keep me amused and make sure I get up in the morning, which helps.

I am very lucky with my family. My mum and dad understand how I feel and take me out every week to make sure I get some fresh air and a different view than my flat. The days out are getting longer as I'm getting better and usually involve a walk with their dogs, as well as lunch and shopping. If I need something heavy or awkward they are happy to take me to get it and are always there if I have a problem.

My parents were especially supportive both financially and emotionally last year when I started having problems with the Benefits Agency. My sick pay had finished and my Incapacity Benefit was stopped as they decided I was well. I put in an appeal and claimed rent and council tax allowance but was left living on about £40.00 a week, which made life very difficult. With help from the Citizens Advice Bureau and the Welfare Rights at Social Services I was successful in my appeal and now have Incapacity Benefit and an Insurance payment from my employers to live on which has made life so much easier.

I enjoy living alone as I feel if I lived with others I would have to make more of an effort to join in and be sociable when I didn't want to be; whereas I can relax and recover as I need to by living alone. At times it is hard work but, thankfully, I have plenty of support.

I am not exactly single from choice nowadays. I had some relationships that didn't work out and felt I was getting a bit old for clubbing so I used to go to the pub with friends. I wasn't looking for a man but wasn't against the idea either. With feeling ill I haven't been able to go out as much and haven't been meeting people. At the moment the thought of starting a new relationship and having to make the effort to get to know someone isn't something I want to do.

In the future, as I get better I would like to meet someone, as I don't want to be alone for the rest of my life wondering what I've missed out on. However, at the moment I'm happy being single and having most of my social life via the computer. This way I don't have to get dressed up to go out, or spend the evening feeling like I'm annoying everyone when I'm tired and can't drink or dance! My way of life suits me and I feel very lucky in being able to live like this. I have had to accept that I have a condition that affects my way of life, and I then had to adapt my life appropriately. I have kept to a simple rule over the years of taking each day at a time.

Fast forward to 2015…

Wow, where do I start? A lot has changed and a lot hasn't, it's fair to say. I was dismissed from my company under the capabilities rule so now I'm unemployed, which is hard to live with. It also means my health insurance ended so now I live on ESA work-related activity group. I lost Mogs but Amber is still very much around and is still keeping me amused.

Due to the bedroom tax I had to move out of my council flat so as I was moving I moved nearer to my parents for mutual support. It means I'm now in a two-up-two-down terrace so have to cope with stairs, but it's a small village where I can walk to the shops or to my parents.

Health-wise it's been good and bad. I developed depression after a bad time that didn't seem to stop so now I have good days and bad days. ME wise I still get the symptoms but I try to manage them better. I don't always succeed but overall it's leveled off.

I've also gained a liver problem, high blood pressure and arthritis, but then that's life not ME I guess.

I'm not able to work but I do voluntary work. I went on an Expert Patient Program course in 2011 and later trained to become a volunteer tutor so now I help run courses. It's hard not to do too much but feeling that I'm able to help people and learn new skills has been fantastic!

It's really helped my confidence levels and I've met new friends. I think it's fair to say that reading back what I wrote in 2002 is slightly shocking and has made me realise just how far I've come and how much life has improved. I'm still single but I have friends and living in a village means I can get out and about so much more. Living nearer my parents means I see them more often and it also means they aren't half an hour away if I'm ill.

Overall it's fair to say life has changed but in a good way. I'm happier than I have been even whilst coping with depression, and I appreciate all that's happened as if I hadn't got ME I wonder if I would have liked the person I was heading to becoming. That work and money obsessed person who never thought of others.

Instead, I value time with people, I love being able to see the countryside and the flowers, I love time with pets. I take time to craft and make cards, do embroidery. Enjoy looking at the beautiful side of life whilst trying not to think of the bad side. It's still there obviously but it's something I can put aside.

It might not be the life I thought I was going to have, but it's a good life.

LIFE WITH *C Henderson*

I hear the sound first. It's a rhythmic whirring, a constant mid-level mechanical hum. I know I am standing in my kitchen but I don't know how I got there. I look down for a clue, a reference point I can clutch for confirmation.

I see that I am wearing my pyjama bottoms with an old sweater and scarf. Fuzzy socks crumple on my feet. It must be morning. I look out of the window to the type of sun that weakly shines in winter. The confident sight fills me with surety. It *is* morning.

The whirring is continuing. It's coming from the grey box in the corner, sitting to one side, occupying a shelf that hangs half way up the wall. I know it's my kitchen wall because I chose the lemon yellow paint that surrounds me. I must be in there to cook breakfast. I sigh with the relief of recognition.

I reach upwards to take a pan out of the cupboard. I don't remember how I know it's there, but my hand touches the long silver handle and I recognise it. A buzz of surety hits again. Some bits of my memory are still working.

When did I arrive in the kitchen? When did I get there? The unlikely inner question turns into a joke at my failures. I snort with laughter. I must have walked there from my bedroom. I thought I was in bed. Yes, I *was* in bed.

From the corner of a picture on the wall I can see my face looking back at me. The side of my face I see in the glass is strange, a shadow of a memory. My hair is shrouding my face with brown marks like streaks of make up after a long night out. In the sudden action of moving my arm, my blurred face looks out with an expression I don't recognise.

Oh, god. Where *did* I go?

I crawled into bed from my bathroom with lead weights on my back and in my bones, wrapped in towels that I have no energy to recall rehanging. The distance crawled with me, inch by inch. I touched the edge of the bed with both hands gratefully and sunk into the bedding with my hair wet and uncaring.

My bed. I went there after I bathed. I've been there since, grasping it's softness like a cradle, sleeping in fitful turns. Endless sleep owns me for hours spiked with gruelling pain.

My mind has been blank since, submerged by nothing, gone nowhere, visiting no-one, absent and foggy like a distant speck on the horizon.

I feel muggy and weak. Exhaustion and sickness encroach in slow segments to occupy me again. The ground lurches under me in a roller coaster dip. I feel it coming and clutch the oven door to stop myself from falling.

The machine pings. I remember the word, it's a microwave! I look inside.

There's food there in a carton. I must have put it in there but I don't remember. I look, and realise it's dinner food.

Where have I gone?

C Henderson

LIFE WITH *Anon*

I was diagnosed with moderate ME approximately three years ago after a virus. I went from being fit and active, able to run 10K without even thinking about it, to having no energy to do the simplest of things.

Throughout it all I managed to work, although I had to drop to part-time and give up any chance of hobbies or a social life. Afternoons, evenings and weekends became recovery time in which to build up energy for the next day of work.

I received several weeks of one-to-one sessions with a specialist, which mainly involved talking and planning strategies. It was great to be believed and taken seriously, yet exhausting having to travel to the sessions, therefore I was secretly glad to be left to cope alone.

I have, however, wrestled with feelings of being given a label and abandoned, as no further help was offered - medical, financial or otherwise, so I have felt compelled to just deal with it.

My condition brings several challenges. Most days, after the slightest exertion, my body screams at me. I use various relaxation techniques to ease the pain. My IBS stops me from enjoying many things other people take for granted, and often prevents me from getting to work on time! Hyperhidrosis, forgetting names and, recently, an extreme loss of balance just add to the fun! Sometimes the coping strategies make everyday life so much extra effort for me, when I have less energy to give than others.

At my worst I can be unable to raise my arms to brush my hair or teeth. At best my lack of muscle strength is laughable. In fact, laughing about it is sometimes the only way to get through! I would like to just wake up one morning and experience normality; the refreshed feeling of having slept instead of the feeling of spending all night in a boxing ring.

I like being told I look well. I know some sufferers don't, but for me this is reassuring. I dislike people thinking I can do all the things normal people do and just get tired a bit quicker - that just shows a total lack of understanding. I have learnt over time it's not worth stressing over people who don't understand, or wasting time trying to explain to those who will never understand. I am very grateful for the close family and friends who do understand; the ones who never let you give up, but let you rest a while when you need to.

Although life has been restricted a lot, I am lucky to have returned to full time work and a few hobbies, including music, which for me is a valuable form of relaxation and achievement. I remain hopeful that my balance issues will pass and I will be able to continue with this. I was once asked why I bothered with hobbies if I was so tired all the time. I think that is maybe one of the most hurtful things anyone has ever said.

I am forever grateful to my husband for going through it all with me and putting up with the extra burden the condition has caused. He has allowed me to have a life and not just an existence throughout it all.

As I await a consultation with a specialist over my recent balance issues I remain hopeful this is just a temporary setback. I still believe I am doing well, recovering as much as possible, and will soon be living life to the full again as far as is possible with such a debilitating condition.

Anon

LIFE WITH *Catherine Humphreys*

As is the situation with so many people, my CFS/ME was triggered by an illness, which in my case was pneumonia and pleurisy.

I ended up being off work from January to the beginning of April last year and, although the illness itself cleared up, I just didn't return to my normal self. The doctor diagnosed me with Post Viral Fatigue Syndrome, which is very common after a long illness, and I was told I should return to normal activity levels soon. However, as time went on, I started to feel worse and developed other symptoms alongside the fatigue; most notably I would continually get headaches, sore throats and ear ache. I had numerous blood tests looking for signs of something lurking in the background, and I even had a couple of appointments with the infectious diseases clinic! The only thing they found was that I was vitamin D deficient.

Between August and the end of November last year I was constantly unwell, picking up something new as soon as I'd just gotten over the last illness, including whooping cough, bronchitis, sinusitis and general colds.

At the end of October, the infectious diseases clinic and my own GP diagnosed CFS/ME and referred me to the clinic in Liverpool. So far I have attended one group session, which was very informative and helped everyone there (sufferers and their partners or parents) understand the condition better and also helped to explain how to manage it as best we could.

We were given a 'starter pack' to go away with to work on, which included sections on managing sleep, rest and relaxation (my biggest problem!), pacing and activity diaries. This has since been followed up with a phone call, which will now lead to attending a couple of workshops on pacing and grading. I think this service will be really helpful in the long run.

The symptoms I personally get are tiredness, weariness, aches and pains in my arms and legs after any activity, 'jelly legs', and I sleep much more than I used to but it's not refreshing, and I fall asleep early on the sofa, at work (occasionally) or even in the cinema from time to time. I have a general feeling of weakness in my limbs or, alternatively, my limbs feel like lead, and I pick up more illnesses and I am ill for longer. I cry A LOT more, I have 'brain fog' – it feels like my brain is wading through treacle and I can't concentrate, and my attention span is miniscule. I sweat after walking short distances, and I have many more symptoms that happen less frequently and consistently but still all add up and put my body through the mill.

I have a mild version of CFS/ME as I do still work full time and I currently commute from Manchester to Liverpool, which gets harder and appears longer every day. However, in order to do this I've had to make some major changes to my life.

Before getting ill I had a fledgling cake business which I've had to totally stop now as I just don't have the energy to work a full day and then come home to start baking and decorating cakes. Just thinking about it just tires me out now! I barely bake anymore, which makes me feel sad as it was something I really enjoyed doing.

My social life has had to be dramatically cut back and it's very rare you'll find me doing anything on a week night. On a weekend I have to put my alarm on and make sure I get up and don't oversleep or I won't be able to get out of bed on a Monday morning.

We try to only do one activity of a weekend and rest and relax for the remainder. My boyfriend has been a huge help in managing the condition with me and he's very supportive and understanding even though it affects his life almost as much as mine. DVD nights have replaced going into town for a meal and drinks – it's a good job we enjoy films so much!

I find limiting my activities one of the hardest things as I've always been a busy person going here, there and everywhere all the time and spending a lot of time with family and friends, which I really miss. I hate telling people I can't plan events in advance as I don't know how I'll feel at the time, which can make everyone's life difficult if definite numbers are needed or deposits etc., or saying I can't do something because I'm tired; it feels like a weak excuse even though I know it's not the same as just needing a bit of extra sleep. I also don't see my parents as often now as I don't have the energy to visit them for dinner on the way home after work. Initially, I felt that resting and relaxing was giving in to the illness but I feel now that I can accept the need to listen to my body as this will help me improve in the long run. It may be some time off but I feel optimistic and hopeful that I will improve; that my symptoms will reduce and my activity levels will get better.

Catherine Humphreys

LIFE WITH *Sharon*

I believe my illness initially began following the sad death of my sister-in-law. She was thirty-nine and diagnosed with breast cancer. She passed away after only four short months after diagnosis. The effect on our family was devastating.

My elderly mum went into depression and I was trying to be the one helping everyone, putting a brave face on all the time, when really, behind the scenes, I was a mess. I couldn't sleep at night, was having mild panic attacks. The number of times I spent the drive into work in floods of tears, then to get there and paint my smile back on as I walked through the door. I was stressed to the limit.

I was backwards and forwards to my GP for a number of things - chest pains, which was believed to be anxiety, panic attacks, and I had a mammogram as I was getting pain in my right breast. Thankfully this was clear. I was never one to see the GP as I was really never ill. I hadn't had a day off work sick for about six years.

I was working full time as a Manager for a large bank, I went swimming at the Gym two or three times a week, ran the house, cooking, cleaning, washing, ironing as well as looking after my two teenage children and running them around to their activities, school etc. I used to do everything, even the decorating. I once decorated our en-suite bathroom between getting home from work one afternoon and cooking the tea. I was non-stop.

Then, I had to stop.

In October 2012 I had quite a stressful experience with a member of my staff. Normally I would handle this type of thing, deal with it and move on, but with the stress I was already under this was too much. We had also bought a puppy in January and, at fifteen weeks old, she broke her leg. This was more stress to deal with. I came down with the flu in February 2013 and never recovered. I was aching all over, exhausted; the pains in my arms, chest and legs were unbelievable and would wake me up in the middle of the night.

Over the next 6 weeks I tried to go into work at least five or six times; each time I lasted about an hour or so, and on the verge of near collapse, had to go home again. I went backwards and forwards to the GP, seeing a different one each time. Each one saying the same thing 'it's a virus and it will work its way out'. It didn't. I was convinced it was more than a virus and suggested maybe I had Chronic Fatigue Syndrome. But no, they wouldn't accept it.

At Easter I managed a full week in work, thinking I was feeling ok, but by Friday I was nearly on my knees again and over the weekend felt dreadful. I finally gave in, went back to see yet another GP and said 'I think I've got Chronic Fatigue'. She agreed! At last! Someone was listening to me after ten weeks of pain and exhaustion.

The GP signed me off work immediately for a couple of weeks and agreed to refer me to the ME/CFS clinic service in Leeds.

I finally got an appointment to see them at the end of June and, with the symptoms I described, coupled with the stress I had been under for the past two years, they diagnosed me at last with ME/CFS. The relief was unbelievable. I wasn't going mad! Someone at last had officially confirmed what I already suspected. I spent the whole of the hour long appointment with the therapist in tears.

My one thought was 'When will I go back to work'. Her reply hit me like a ton of bricks, 'Don't even think about work until you can manage day to day life', she said. But working meant I was well, and back to normal. How could I not go back? And as soon as possible?

I quickly came to realise that work was not a possibility. Doing housework was not a possibility. Normal life was not a possibility.

My partner had to take over the general cleaning, cooking and washing duties as I just couldn't function. The pain I got after any type of activity was unbelievable. I spent the days crashed on the sofa. I was managing to take the kids to school in the mornings and walk the dog for 10 minutes or so but that was about it. I remember driving to school one afternoon with excruciating pain in my left shoulder, and when my son got in the car I just burst into tears. I was in agony.

I finally gave in and got a cleaner, as working and trying to run the house was getting too much for my partner too, and, let's face it, men just don't clean the same, do they! When I was well I vowed I wouldn't have a cleaner, I could do it all myself couldn't I? I now wish I had got one years ago! There are lots of things in hindsight that I wish I had done - got a cleaner, cut my hours at work, and got a decorator in. But hindsight is such a wonderful thing.

My second visit to the clinic, about six weeks later, was one where my illness was quickly put into perspective. We now had to look at how I was going to move forward to recover. Again I spent the hour in tears. It was tough facing up to the reality that your life has suddenly changed so dramatically. I had to now learn to stop, slow down completely and to say No! Something I had never really done.

The Therapist started off by giving me some activity charts to complete and I had to do these hour by hour, colour coding low activity, high activity and rest periods. She wanted to have at least three hour periods a day! This was completely alien to me. I rested when I went to bed, or in the evening when I sat and watched TV. But this was to be complete rest, away from everything.

I had already started to put some things in place for myself by walking the dog every day to make sure I got some exercise, as it was the only thing I could do. I started off at about five minutes a day.

I had warm relaxing baths in the evening and a lie down for half an hour afterwards. But the activity I was doing in between was along the lines of 'push and crash'. When I felt well I was going hell for leather doing stuff and then I would be in pain and crash afterwards. I had to learn to pace myself.

I found an app for my phone that was really for Fibromyalgia sufferers to use to record their activity and pain levels during the day, but I adapted this to record mine. It was interesting to see and track how activity affected me, and by monitoring this I learnt how to slow myself down and do less. It was encouraging to then track how my pain diminished in line with slowing down and introducing relaxation into my routine.

I had been back to the GP for something for the pain and after trying Amitriptyline, which made me feel worse and like a zombie; I prescribed myself Arnica, which is a homeopathic herbal pain relief. And it worked!

I spent most of my days researching ME/CFS and the symptoms, causes and possible cures, and what worked for some and what didn't. I would try anything if I thought it would help. I researched what supplements to take that would help and started to practice guided meditation, and saw quite a big reduction in my pain. I took the time out mid-morning and late afternoon to do forty-five minutes of meditation every day, with a further thirty minutes after my bath in the evening. It took discipline and routine but I have always liked routine.

I also started having fortnightly aromatherapy massages to relieve my stress and found a fantastic massage therapist who lived locally. She also did Reiki so I had a few sessions of those too and was amazed at some of the results. I began to establish a baseline – this is an amount of activity you can easily cope with in a day that does not leave you feeling exhausted at the end of it and in pain.

This takes weeks to get to if not months and is a slow arduous task: One day you might feel better than the day before and the temptation is to do more, but you then pay for it later. It took me about three months to get a good baseline in place. The key is to feel fine whilst you're sat about doing nothing. Once you feel like that you can then start to build up gradually, bit by bit.

At first I could only manage a short walk in the park around the small pond and that would be it. I would then come home and spend the rest of the morning on the sofa watching TV with meditation in between. But slowly, over time, my activity levels increased and I built up my dog walks to thirty minutes each morning, and I introduced other things such as positive visualisation and EFT.

I got to where I could do the usual school runs and walk the dog and do a bit of shopping or meet up with a friend for coffee for an hour or so as well. At weekends, I started to go into the local town and do some shopping with my mum and daughter and we would have coffee in a café. I would drive down and back. This was after about five or six months of pacing and finding my baseline. I then introduced some gentle stretches and exercises in the evening to my routine.

Every small step is a milestone to someone with ME/CFS and is a positive indication that recovery is slowly taking place. It can take months and months to move even one minute forward in how long you can sustain something. One thing the illness certainly teaches you is patience in bucketfuls. Something I never had much of when I was ever ill before. I always used to say I hadn't time to be ill. Now I have to make time to be ill and lots of it.

I still have a long way to go in my recovery and am at present about 75% housebound, but progress is progress.

Sharon

LIFE WITH *Dyson by Dyson's Nanny*

Dyson is fifteen years old now and is a funny, bright, intelligent, articulate and, once, very sociable young lad. He has wisdom beyond his years, watches tons of documentaries and has an opinion on just about everything! We live in Ireland.

When he was twelve years of age Dyson was struck down with a viral illness (we now know it was Epstein Barr virus) in April 2012. He was very ill with it. His GP didn't know what was wrong with him and he wasn't sent for any blood tests. After a few weeks of being really ill, the virus seemed to attack his respiratory system and he developed a viral pneumonia. While he was trying to recover from that he woke up one morning covered in chicken pox.

His system had basically undergone an all-out viral attack. He eventually recovered enough to get back to school and we thought we had put it all behind us. Looking back on it now, however, it was clear that he wasn't 100% that summer.

He managed to still do all the normal things he loved like swimming, cycling, hill walking, going to the gym, playing table tennis, diving, etc but he did seem a little more 'sedate' than normal. I just thought he was 'growing up' and was leaving some of the exuberance of youth behind him.

He started his second level school in September 2012 – something he had looked forward to for months and months on end. He loved the idea of becoming grown up and independent and his best friend had also got a place in the same school. Life was good.

After two weeks in school he came home one day and almost collapsed on the floor. I'll never forget how ill he looked. There were tears in his eyes as he said how awful he felt. That night he started vomiting and then went on to have severe diarrhoea. Life was never the same after that day. He simply never recovered.

I use that date, 8th September 2012, as the defining moment of the onset of his illness but, truly, perhaps it was brewing since the previous April when he had all those viral illnesses in succession. Who knows? And that is exactly the problem....who knows?

The medical profession likes it if you get sick and then they treat you and then you get better. They're not so happy with you if you get sick, then they treat you and then you don't get better. I think it makes them uncomfortable. In fact I always think back to that first bout of sickness he got and the many trips to his GP. At one point the GP said to him 'you make me feel like I can't doctor'. I suppose at least she was honest.

Dyson's presentation in September 2012 included severe stomach issues, which didn't resolve for two years despite numerous hospital admissions, medications, other interventions, surgical biopsies, various tests, etc. His bowels had completely stopped working from November of that year. The hospital tried everything in their armour, but nothing worked. We even considered a stoma but pulled back from this because of the long term implications and complications.

Eventually, something very simple and natural worked for him. A remedy I got from a person I never met in real life but met on an internet forum – a lifesaver for me. So far he has been five months free of the bowel issues and we are keeping our fingers crossed.

Although all his hospital admissions related to his bowel issues, he also had this myriad of debilitating symptoms that were, at best, being studiously 'ignored' by the hospital and, at worst, being challenged by some ignorant members of his Consultant team.

In fairness to his consultant, he did diagnose him with a Post Viral Illness at the time and predicted a prolonged recovery. This has since been confirmed as ME by Dr. Nigel Speight. It was the consultant who discovered the Epstein Barr Virus in Dyson's system. However it was also the same consultant who immediately referred him to the Psychiatric Service in the hospital and never inquired about his other symptoms since! Talk about washing your hands of the problem!

We were never told what to expect. We were never told about any symptoms. We were left to muddle along and crash and burn to our hearts content. We were left in the hands of a psychiatrist who had misinterpreted the referral and believed that what he was dealing with was a child who had school avoidance issues.

I ended up making an official complaint to the hospital, calling a care plan meeting and bringing the teams together so that we could sort the mess out. We did - and then the psychiatrist left and was replaced with someone who could just have easily come straight out of the Wessely School. She recommended putting Dyson, a thirteen year old happy go-lucky, sick kid, on Prozac because (in her words) 'she wasn't happy that he wasn't getting better'. The more I write about this, the more furious I get. Needless to say I took him out of that service.

So just in case you were wondering what are these symptoms that Prozac was supposed to help – read on. If you have ME, look away now, because you will probably be bored with this already!

If you haven't got ME or don't know someone who has, stick with it because you might learn something. He had a 24/7 headache in his right temple, tinnitus, balance problems, nosebleeds, light sensitivity, deteriorating eyesight, temperature dysregulation, complete sleep reversal, bone and muscle pain, inability to generate energy, complete exhaustion, cognitive problems including the inability to process simple instructions, short-term memory loss, new onset dyslexia, the inability to retain information, sensitivity to noises, nausea, vomiting, regular swollen and painful glands, heartburn, rashes and bowel dysfunction.

To his eternal credit, when Dyson heard that she wanted to put him on Prozac, he looked her directly in the eye and said 'Will it help the pain in my arse?' That was a defining moment in his journey of self-advocacy!

This is a short version of Dyson's journey with ME. We are into year three now and we are hoping and praying for a treatment or a cure. He still hasn't made it back to school and every day is a challenge. Each day is filled with pain, exhaustion and a host of other nasties.

I just also want to say that I have made so many friends through the ME Facebook groups and other ME forums and I thank each and every one of you for making this journey a little bit more bearable. We would be totally lost with you all.

Dyson by Dyson's Nanny

LIFE WITH *Germaine Hypher*

The Naming of the Shrewd

My name is Esmé. In truth, I have no name but all things must be called to account. Maybe when they identify me they'll know how to handle me. They'll call Rumpelstiltskin to my wild dance and control my fevered flinging's. Until then it's up to me to name myself and find what power lies here. It's strange to refer to *myself* when I'm so used to identifying with my host.

I'm not proud of what I am. Is that where her illegitimate self-doubts emanate from? Is my influence more pervasive then either of us realised? If so then maybe I've found my story. I've titled myself (Esmé. I like it.) But what is a title without a tale? *She* could be my story. *She* knows her name but so often it's the wrong one — all hunchback letters squatting in a disgruntled huddle and so much confusion over their sound. It's all crashing consonants and mistaken identities and where's the power in that? So we're a fractured pair, she and I, knitting some kind of narrative together and neither of us knowing where to cast off.

Inherited memory is a slippery enemy, especially when many don't even believe an infectious agent like me could master such a skill. I've bugged the past, wrapped my wet coils around her, and set myself to replay. Looping like a Mobius strip, my miasma and I travel the circuit of a one-armed swimmer round and around her body, deep in the brine of her being, playing with the coral of her muscles. I dart through the flickering neon of her deep-sea synapses and cling like a barnacle to her organs and glands. I don't want her to suffer but if I don't do this then I am nothing. And we must all exist to add a new perspective to the tale. Maybe one day she'll tell hers. Here I am finally voicing mine and I find she's competing for lead role. I never considered that when I named myself.

Esmé. I like it.

But where do I start? I know I'm just a paragraph in a persistent script. I'll start with what I know, and I know she would have run barefoot through waves with her laughter swooped on by gulls and carried off like stolen chips to be devoured by the wind if I'd have let her. I know she'd have lost herself in forests and an artist's picture of the world. I also know she found far more than she bargained for because of me. The canopy of woodlands is an open sky compared to where I led her.

'So where did you take her? Who are you?' Oh reader, if only the answer were as easy as the question. My viral pathway is a serpentine route, pebbled with all the deception and desire of Eden's own snake.

I took her from the swings with her eight-year-old friends, face painted like a Native American warrior, pushing the limits of gravity until she felt sick with giddy laughter, and I grabbed that nausea; I nurtured it, took it under one arm, her under the other, and I ran. I turned up the playground sounds until her head hurt then I'd keep her awake with the volume inside. Sleep deprivation is a powerful ally but you have to know how to use it.

Let her drift and doze, believing day and night that she can't stay awake, but keep the plasma screen in her head on at all times. Keep the rapid eye movement flickering insanely, turn up the mayhem, and while she's dreaming her way through a twelve-hour night, her body's still at work. She'll wake with coddled confusion and brittle abilities but will never guess at the game.

She wasn't easy — didn't lie with illness without encouragement. I stroked her skin until the shiver of invisible fingers weakened her and persuaded her she was mine. I stalked her when she walked with her parents, taking her body, the path, the smell of life for granted. I watched and I began sapping her strength with my need. I spied her at nine on the sheepskin rug, her personal stage, twisting and shimmying for the music in the room and the spotlight in her head, and I pulled the rug from under her. Watched her legs buckle and her eyes blank out the facts. I saw her get up and start again, and I kept vigil over her muscles' malpractice as she walked to school and tried to escape.

She thought if she kept moving I couldn't catch her. I helped her run through the degenerative years straight into my arms. I wore her down until, when she finally succumbed, it was me she turned to. Oh, she may have laid her aching head on her mother's lap and entrusted her body to the adults around her, but it was me she let in. Me she allowed to teach her about herself. It was my advice she listened to and my scrambled suggestions of pain and persistence.

'Don't give up! Don't give in! Go, go, go! Push through!' Her nature was strong. How else could we have worked so well together? Her obstinate refusal to step down from life and float on the waves of weakness were exactly what I required. I could hold her hand and lead her through my maze without her ever stopping to question. She would keep walking, keep talking, keep moving those dreams from her head to her days, pushing and pulling them into physical reality for me to catch hold of like a tenacious puppy and wrench from her grasp. She held tight, I'll give her that. Eventually, between us, we had torn them into ragged remnants, jagged seams separating and gaping at their own inadequacy.

Another person may have heeded common sense, may have stood back and looked at the situation, rested a weary body in the grip of collapse and taken time out to outwit the insurgent within. But she fought fire with fire and I won. So I say, anyway. And I've said it often enough for her to believe it.

I drop reminders of how other bodies function. Give her just enough hope and semblance of normality to egg her on, lead her into thinking she could fight me off if only she had the ingenuity or the tenacity. So now she has guilt and shame to add to the arsenal against her own body.

Her legs may no longer run but I know how to keep her racing. Adrenaline on overflow so that her pulse races, her thoughts race, her speech speeds up and her enthusiasms chase her fears, outrun them at times only to bring her down like a gazelle with the lion of exhaustion on its back.

'Fight or flight,' I whisper. 'Fight or flight.' And she can't fight me so she runs inside her head. Runs through her options, her hopes, her inadequacies; running on empty until her body is run down beyond despair. And there I have her. There I find myself.

'Push, push, push. Don't go. Stop. Go. Stop!' Oh, the alphabetti-spaghetti messages I feed her! Pull her on to knock her back and her body is a confusion of overexertion, under-performance and messed up neurology. Don't get me wrong, I'm no head-fuck. I'm just doing what I must. Evolutionary biology doesn't spend centuries mastering something like me to waste me on the weakest. It siphons me through bloodlines and bit-part existences until it locates the right time and place. It finds willpower, determination, dysfunctional dreams, crippled ancestry and enough stressors to weaken, weaken, weaken. What would be the point in gripping the body of a melancholic couch-hugger? Some of my brethren do, I know. A host is a host to some, I guess. But she and I are more similar than she cares to imagine. I need a challenge. It strengthens me.

I've got next generations to think of too, you know. She thinks it's all about her. She doesn't have a clue.

As for her selfish claim on the suffering I inflict, it hasn't occurred to her yet that I *am* her pain. When she feels it, that's all I am. When she pushes it to the edge of her experience, attempting to ignore my call, I still lurch from spasmodic twist to heaving morass of hormonal fluctuation. Thud, tug, rip, blaze in a tempest of opposition. It's what I am.

She spins with sickening vertigo while flat on her back and considers the fairness and ferocity of life. Does she once consider the fairness of my life — the constant effort it takes to derail her complex organism just so that I have a home?

Her temperature swoops, taunting her skin into a contradiction of Goosebumps and clammy slip-slide, extremities cracking under the pressure of juvenile chilblains. Fatigue pulls like quicksand, sucking at her personality until she can't lift her head above the silt. Her lymphatic system clogs with the by-products of living so that drainage is impaired and muscles burn with the post-marathon throb of minimal movement. Have you ever watched a bandy-legged long-distance runner after they've hit 'the wall', limbs swinging offbeat, wobbling spectacularly prior to collapse? Imagine that not confined to legs but throughout the system, visible, invisible. Here now, now gone. And back again. Imagine hitting the wall daily. That's what I am. I'm the brick wall and the smack that rebounds off it, hovering hysterically in the air before falling with the victim to sink, sink, sink ...

I know how to wear a body down. It hurts, but I'm no martyr. It builds me up — reinforces what I am. All those symptoms in a symphony of pseudo-control and her body thinks it's gaining on me but I've pulled the ultimate trick. Turned its combat on itself. Her brain jams under the pressure of too many neurons firing blindly, over-absorbing light, sound, touch, imaginings and reality. She shakes in the presence of movement as her body struggles to identify messages from her environment and the concept of energy, but she forgets that I have to surrender myself in that moment to actually be the tumult of shivering muscles.

Not just the ones people notice, either, but all the hidden musculature that supports her internal organs and the movement of eyeballs; her ability to inflate lungs and widen a jaw enough to yawn. Ha! I've worked on that one, too. Limit the passage of oxygen through cell walls and where's the body going to source its vital life-support from? She can deep breathe, chakra breathe, clamp her face with an oxygen mask if she wants. It's not going to help. Oh, there's enough passing through to maintain the illusion of functionality. I've got it sorted. I know what I'm doing.

She berates herself for immobility and dependence. Never mind *changing* the world, she just wants to be a *part* of it. Fool! She can't see that she *is* experiencing it, only not in the way she'd expected. And as for feeling inert — God, if she only knew the work that goes on inside of her ...

She has no idea of the labour I put myself to, the hormones I dictate to and the systems I infiltrate. But hardest of all is the secrecy. A grey pallor sometimes threatens to give me away, along with occasionally slurred speech, but the palpitations and difficulty breathing can be passed off as hysteria so I don't concern myself much with those. The mayhem let loose by the flood of cortisol in her blood appears psychological and as for memory loss, well, most onlookers claim they know what that's like anyway. (As if their forgetfulness stretches to a daily forgetting of loved ones' names or substitution of 'potato' for 'pillowcase' because the brain thought alliteration might mask meltdown.

Give me *some* credit.). No, I don't get caught out often. But it's hard work being suffering itself and still managing to cover your tracks.

Some see through my disguises. They hear me whispering through weakened vocal chords or lurking behind her eyes, but no one's traced me yet. It's an art, you know. I used to see it as survivalism; now it's a vocation. Not one on which you can proudly wax lyrical over a smooth Merlot at dinner parties admittedly, but I've learnt not to play with pride and dinner parties aren't an issue when suppression is your bedfellow. Occupation isn't a job; it's a military term.

I've come to know every aspect of this home intimately. I befriended and sidled up to her inner system, acquainted myself so naturally that it soon forgot I wasn't from these parts. I penetrated its codes and played with its patterns. A few tweaks here, a chromosomal nudge there, a little genetic material mingled with my own and I'd perpetuated my own existence, transducing and mutating my way into a fixed abode. That's got to be an achievement, for a squatter.

Credit where credit's due, she's worked hard at evicting me. Pediatricians and poultices, faith healers and consultants, prescriptions and potions. Even spells and psychology. But how do you expel what you can't find? They can work on the mess I've made, clear up some of the detritus, but while they can't see me or my point of entry, it's impossible to push me out. And as for the ones who don't even accept that I'm here — see her as a weakened mind creating her own poltergeist — no chance. I win hands down.

But it's changing. It's not as easy as it used to be. Decades drip by and I do my work but so do the others. More people recognise me than used to and intelligent minds hear of my presence.

I'm not the only one who likes a challenge. They're on my tail. None of them know my name though, and for that reason I know I've time yet. I can still shape-shift with the best of diseases and lead a dappled dance of decay. I'm not naive; I know they'll name me one day. They always do.

But there's time yet and, just like her, I'm not giving up without a fight.

So that's our story. Or some fragmented part of it filtered through me for want of one all to myself. Even if I rest for a time, am caught up with or called by name and she begins to pay less attention to my part in our tale, she'll never be fully free. We've shared too much for the ripples to smooth out and lay a sheen over our past. Her cells have archived our memories and her genes have handed them down.

Even as I may dream and scheme in dormancy, responses and patterns have been shaped like a marble run for her to roll along.

She may not know my name but I am Esmé.

© *Germaine Hypher*

This story first appeared in the anthology *Sunshine In A Bag.* For more info, please visit http://brigitsquill.wordpress.com

Germaine Hypher

LIFE WITH *Donna Anstead*

My story begins in 1992. I am fefteen years old and have spent the last year or so with what the doctors called recurring glandular fever. I have had to quit the school hockey team and leave my role as a court judge in the annual school production. Some weeks I manage a day or so or half a day at school. All my friends but one have slowly drifted away from me.

I am lonely, becoming depressed and despondent. I had always wanted to be a teacher, now I am struggling with my GCSE coursework as I am so vacant and exhausted. I don't recall at what stage it was decided that I had ME. I do recall being sent to RAF Halton to see a specialist who was pioneering hyperbaric oxygen treatment for ME, in the hope that the pure oxygen would help sufferers feel better. I had to go to this pressurised chamber for an hour a day every day for a month. I hated it, apart from the fact that I had to try to go out every day and my poor mum had to come home early from work to take me, it was excruciatingly painful, the pressure on my swollen glands and ears was horrific. To top it off I felt no benefit what so ever.

The next year or so went by in a blur; I remember lying on the sofa in my pjs day and night as I couldn't get upstairs. Sometimes I couldn't eat with the mess my throat was in, drinking was almost as bad. I learned about my old friends from school via my sister and my one remaining friend.

I recall being particularly upset at finding out a boy I used to like was going out with someone! It didn't really make much difference, I had hardly been at school for two years, he probably didn't know who I was, but I was still gutted. I also remember feeling not so bad around Christmas and deciding I was going to blooming well go out! By the time I had bathed and got ready I was in so much pain and so exhausted that I curled up on my bedroom floor and cried after sending my sister and friend out without me.

On the odd occasion I made it to school, teachers were quick to tell me I was doing a great job of 'swinging the lead' and 'pulling the wool over mum's eyes'. This really hurt me. Some teachers even refused my medical certificates which were to be entered with my coursework.

When I was seventeen I started to get longer and longer spells of being ok. Eventually I was up to getting an apprenticeship as a dental nurse. I had a few setbacks but got through them and my life moved on - I wasn't half the person I was before I was ill, but I was coping.

Time passed, I met my husband and had two daughters; I was low energy generally, but fine. By 2007 I was able to run in 10k runs, I lifted weights, and was self-employed as a child-minder. Unfortunately, the running caused the cartilage to tear in both my knees and I needed surgery. This was 2009 and the beginning of an ME relapse.

To cut a long story short, I was back to the pathetic crying, ill, energy-less mess that I had been all those years ago. I had to leave my part time job; the GP I had now didn't believe in ME and said I was depressed and put me on antidepressants. I felt so guilty for being a rubbish mum and useless as a wife, friend, sister, daughter. I was in so much pain, losing days to brain fog and exhaustion, and saw no end in sight. I was so indignant that this was happening to me again! And felt as though my life had been ruined again. Time went by and I slowly had longer spells of feeling ok. Eventually, I felt well enough to go back to work for a few hours a week. I was at a management stage; I had to gauge on a daily basis how much I could do.

I restricted any 'unnecessary' activities like socialising, expending of energy etc. and, by early 2013, I was working three days a week. I spent this year being positive and saying that I didn't have ME, I had had ME but I was over it and going to get better and better, like before. I took meditation classes and became qualified as a Reiki practitioner. By the Oct 2013 I was really feeling the strain, having a lot of time off work and getting worried that I seemed to be getting worse and not better. I decided after a lot of soul searching that I would leave my job and become self-employed with my Reiki - this was in Jan 2014.

I showed little improvement over the coming months, but with my reduced activity I wasn't any worse. By Sept 2014 I had enrolled on a complimentary therapy course at college and was looking forward to (and hoping I would cope with) learning Swedish massage, aromatherapy and reflexology.

By October I had already been off sick at least once a week, by early November I had had several chest infections and pneumonia. Cue relapse. I attended college irregularly; until the Christmas holidays over which I made the divesting choice to quit and just do a four hour a week reflexology course instead. So, here I am in 2015, so far I have managed to attend that four hour session twice, college have been very good and understanding and my new GP actually believes in ME, although he prefers to call it CFS…he is referring me to CFS services.

I spend a lot of my time in bed, rarely asleep just lying like a vacant zombie log thing. Sometimes I do the sofa, but that causes pain. I cry almost daily, I think I am grieving for the life I wanted, the life I planned. I berate myself for not being up to doing things, for being a burden and a waste of space. This is where I am now, waiting to be seen by CFS service; I have applied for a blue badge and PIP. I didn't want to, it makes me feel ashamed and like a malingerer.

I don't know if I am going to get better, so I try my best to make the most of what I've got. I am grateful for having a supportive and understanding family; they make my life more tolerable.

Donna Anstead

LIFE WITH *Coleen Mackenzie*

Awake am I, I do not know? BUT then the shutters start to rise! Giving me a misty view of the room, I hear voices in the distance, what can I do?

My body is still, my mind alert, I want to join in, yet I feel I am not really here?

The shutters close quickly and silence surrounds me.

The shutters begin to rise again; I strain to see clearly to find a clear space…within this foggy cloud.

The voices are louder; I want to be there - for I recognise friends, grandchildren, my family, my husband…OH! Let me share in the fun, so I push myself forward to search amongst the mist, to find that step onward, to take me through the mist. But wait!

My body feels heavy, my heads a lead weight. It feels like I've a back pack filled with jagged stones, jarring on my body, creating aches and pains around my shoulders, my neck… Every movement the back pack gets tighter and my neck begins to cease. Still, I have expectations of myself. For I am the life and sole of the party. I am an independent woman. I love my Family!

So come on Girl … (My head still works if the rest of me does not) so I roll myself forward and try to get to my feet, they are cold, solid and lifeless, - This is not who I am??!! I feel for the floor as my body tries to co-ordinate my movements and thoughts…Then it happens. A moment of 'clear thinking' and I say boldly 'enough is enough!' I Demand of me to stand! And walk as if I were FREE.

But the weight pulls me backwards, and I find myself lying on a bed, staring at the ceiling, I feel heavy to move. Somehow it's not like I'm in my body for sure, for this back pack carries more than I know? Hello! I'm full of fun! But this bag is a burden; it has me cased in the unknown. I'm waning…but still fighting - Who am I and what is happening? With exhaustion Nothing to do now but be still! – I wish to be the - me I know - and get up and go!

But the shutters close down fast, just as I hear a voice clearly…but I cannot reply?

But my bodies not willing although I want my voice to let go.

Time is irrelevant now and so it goes on; I want to get out of this pain and mist. But the time it keeps passing and the days they do too.

I don't realise often the passing of time, but I am aware there are days that go by, do not ask me the day of the week or what year, or ask me a question, It shakes me with fear and often with unease. My work before could see me no glum as I would challenge all and everyone.

But where I am Now? For, I do not know? I cannot control my 'sleeping' I cannot take, the pressure of uncertainty…of when I'm awake Is this a mistake? So Assertive I was? And I realise that there's something ticking within me - a different clock.

The shutters won't open and I can't go through the veil

I'm not who I used to be? **The** woman running her own business, workshops and events, loving her grandchildren and working with her horses.

I have my own expectations of who I am…..I thought that - is what I have to do! Run the shop Create workshops redesign modules, be with my horses, do the housework, books, simple things like have the grandkids every other weekend, and visit my family…I loved every minute of that. Then suddenly it was all taken away, it was like ME/Fibromyalgia Imploded in me over night! And EVERYTHING was stripped away!

My Shop - CLOSED, (My Beloved) Horses - REHOMED, Grandchildren - Couldn't stay over.

I was Empty, I could not stay Awake, My head and body could not deal with any form of stress or trauma?

Today!!!!! Five years on I have gone from being bedbound and being awake for a mere two hours a day, sporadically, to eat and go to the bathroom.

I am in my fifties now; I'm a granny and a whole life ahead of me so I woke the other morning with the idea that this is my life now! I am not who I was?

So every day now is a challenge. I Enjoy the moment of being awake for what it is.. I may have four hours in a day now, more or less… But it is what I do with that moment that counts, not reminiscing of my past. But enjoying the moment for NOW… and blessing what I can do instead of what I cannot…

Coleen Mackenzie

LIFE WITH *Karen*

I became ill in 1996, just before my thirty-second birthday, after yet another 'virus' to which I seemed susceptible, as I had them regularly throughout my twenties. I thought this would be like the others, weak and ill, but gone in a couple of weeks. Unfortunately, I was wrong.

I was a mature, Post-Graduate student at this time, living in Bristol. I loved my studies although didn't know where it would lead me in my career. I had worked in an office as a secretary prior to returning to full-time education when I was twenty-six. Apart from 'viruses' and IBS, I was reasonably healthy and able to live a 'normal' life, socialising and working hard. When I became ill in March 1996 I thought I'd recover in the Easter holidays and return to finish my studies. I had had a bad cold, become ill whilst driving home from Bristol, recovered, and, two weeks later, become ill again.

The doctor said it was a virus and then post-viral fatigue; antidepressants were offered which made me groggy. I was exhausted, sleeping a lot, unable to concentrate, not able to think clearly, weak and nauseous, but I didn't need antidepressants and expected to eventually bounce back. I managed, with my mum's help, to attend the last few days of my course as much of the work was done and attendance was no longer necessary. I had a placement in Cardiff, but lasted only half a day before the pain kicked in. I didn't know what was happening to me.

I seem to remember that it was mum who saw a leaflet for an ME local group, to which we went. I was upset afterwards as everyone there had been ill for such a long time and I couldn't imagine that kind of life. Mum reassured me that the ones who had recovered wouldn't go anymore. I got in touch with a chap who was ill who told me about a consultant at Nottingham City Hospital; I went to see him and he diagnosed Post-Viral Fatigue. I also found out that Dr Myhill held a clinic near to my parents once a month and so went along to see her. She did lots of tests and recommended B12 and Magnesium injections. She suspected Gilberts Syndrome and diagnosed ME. No-one seemed to have any concrete answers.

My mum was so helpful and supported me all she could. It is frightening when you don't know what is happening to you or why; especially when the doctors are clueless and there seem no answers. I was sleeping a lot, felt very weak, nauseous and achy. I joined lots of the ME charities in a bid for answers and began writing to other single people in a similar situation to myself.

Through this I 'met' Mike, a fellow ME sufferer who lived in Wales, and we corresponded and spoke on the phone when we could. We got together very quickly in October 1997 as we couldn't get to know each other in the usual way, but began living together and have been together pretty much ever since.

In 2001 Dr Myhill found that I had problems with my thyroid and I was put on thyroxine (50mcg). I thought this may be the answer to my health problems but, sadly, it was not. Mike and I got married in a small, short ceremony in May 2001 – not exactly what I would have chosen but all we could manage within our limitations. We continued to search for answers and undertook many tests, privately and through the NHS, but nothing really came of it. I was found to have positive ANA and Smooth Muscle antibodies, as well as abnormal LFTs but doctors didn't know what to make of it and could offer nothing.

In 2005 I became even worse, and thought I was having an ME relapse. I struggled for five months before paying to see an Endocrinologist who prescribed T3, and told me to increase my T4 as ME sufferers tend to do better when their T4 levels are at the top end of the range. I gradually did that and feel, since then, that I have become much more stable, without the awful 'relapses' and 'viruses' I endured for months previously. I wish my doctor had told me to increase my thyroxine and that staying on 50mcg for four years was not a good idea but that it would need eventually to be increased.

I can't begin to explain how difficult life is having ME. I have lost so much of my life – the chance to have children, a career, travel and to socialise - the limitations are enormous; as well as the illness robbing me of strength and confidence. Yet I continue to try to stay positive and look at what I have rather than I have not. There are so many others who are so much worse than me and I try always to remember that. I can read a little more now than I used to be able to; I do what I can on a daily basis, staying within my limitations as much as possible.

I think one of the worst aspects of having ME, apart from feeling so ill and there being no cure, is the attitude of doctors and the general public to it. ME sufferers would just like some acknowledgement of the struggles they face and not to be thought of as malingerers or psychologically ill; nor is it a lifestyle choice. I don't know when this will change but it has to be for progress to be made in finding a cure for this devastating illness which blights so many lives.

Karen

LIFE WITH *Claire*

I had a really lovely childhood. And by seventeen, my life was all mapped out. I had passed my GCSEs with nine A*s, I was on for four As at A-level, had managed to secure a place at Oxford University, and I had a busy social life, including swimming seven times a week! I had worked since I was fourteen, first in a chip shop, then in a sports shop, and most recently as a lifeguard. I loved my life, I was dating and I had lots and lots of friends.

At first I just had flu-like symptoms, for around seven weeks, which seemed to clear up, but, a couple of months later, I got sick and didn't recover. There then followed many, many doctor appointments, between which I was in bed. Asleep. I slept between eighteen and twenty hours a day. And when I was awake I was a zombie, in a bubble of aches and pains and depression. I was so bad I didn't see my life slowly disappearing, until I had very few friends, no place at university, no qualifications, and a family so scared and bewildered they didn't know what would be waiting for them whenever they got home.

Gradually I became better at managing my symptoms, and, with a very early diagnosis (a rarity in 2000, when very few doctors even recognised the existence of ME), I began to try to piece my life back together, taking medication for the pain and the depression, and having weekly lymphatic massages and physiotherapy.

My mum read every book she could on the condition, and my father, who has his own health problems, rubbed my back and understood how horrendous it was for me to slowly watch my old life slip away. My sister, who I shared a room with, used to keep me company at nights, and my two brothers tried to do everything they could to keep me company, to make me comfortable, and to keep my spirits up.

I eventually returned to college, but it was almost impossible to attend most days, and I was so angry about all I had lost I could barely focus on rebuilding my life.

I am so glad, though, that when I first got sick I had no idea what having ME truly involved. I have had a number of miscarriages, due to my inability to support a growing child within my body. I ache from head to toe all the time. I have bad depression (leading me to attempt suicide), and I suffer from panic attacks, and acute anxiety. I have poor circulation, and my immune system is all but useless. I have headaches that make light almost unbearable. I get shooting pains throughout my body, and I have problems with my heart.

At thirty-two, I have now had ME for fifteen years. I had good periods, when I could work, and I managed to move away from Bury, where I grew up, to attend Loughborough University. But halfway through my second year I had a massive relapse and have never recovered from this.

However, just before this relapse I met the most amazing man, my now husband, Guy. When I got sicker, he left his job, took a much lower paid position, relocated across the country, and we moved in together so he could take care of me. He is the best thing that has ever happened to me, and whenever the devastation of all I have lost, and the depression threatens to overtake me, and the longing for the life I feel I should have had becomes too strong, I remember that without falling ill I would never have found him.

My life now involves lots of resting, lots of pain, lots of sleep, but 2015 finds me much more able to manage my condition, with careful planning and finally a good balance of medication (Gabapentin, Lemotrogine, Quetiapine, Buspirone, Codeine, Paracetamol, etc.), and I am halfway through an accountancy degree, in the hope that I can work from home at some point in the future.

I have loyal and understanding friends, who understand my illness, and do anything they can to help me, and accommodate my limitations. My husband and I have no money, very few possessions, and we lurch from disaster to disaster – mostly due to drama with my condition – but we have so much fun! We laugh all the time, and (corny I know!) he makes it better!

My aunt (who died last year) once gave me a lovely analogy which now provides the framework by which I live my life now.

Once when we were talking about how sad I was about all I have lost, she said: *'Imagine that you were on a plane to Italy. You have packed for the weather, you have learned the language, you have planned your itinery and you are really excited. And then the plane touches down and you are in Norway. You can't speak the language, your wardrobe is wrong, and you can't see the things you wanted, or have the experiences you were looking forward to, with the people you were expecting to spend your time with. But that doesn't mean Norway doesn't have things to offer. It's not how you imagined, and you have to adjust your expectations, but you can either rail against the unfairness of it all, or try to be positive.'*

Claire

Thank you to everyone who has contributed, and all who have read this. Your purchase supports vital bio-medical research by Invest In ME.

www.investinme.org.uk

ABOUT THE AUTHOR

Hayley Green is an ME sufferer based in the UK. Previous publications include *101 Tips For Coping With ME, Understanding ME – A Guide For Friends, Family & Carers and What is ME? A Guide For Children.*

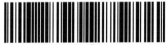

Printed in Great Britain
by Amazon